ADVANCE PRAISE

Dr. Deana Murphy gets it! *Lead2Flourish* is at the cutting edge of leadership development. Dr. Murphy helps us understand that to transformationally elevate as a leader, we need to (1) awaken to our ego-related fears that dictate our leadership at an unconscious level (recognize), (2) heal from our ego-related fears (renovate & rebuild), and (3) step out as a value-creating leader (recharge). *Lead2Flourish* walks us through this process in a way that is sure to help you elevate your ability to become a greater positive influence within your spheres of responsibility.

—**RYAN GOTTFREDSON, PhD**, LEADERSHIP PROFESSOR AT CALIFORNIA STATE UNIVERSITY-FULLERTON, AND AUTHOR OF THE WALL STREET JOURNAL AND USA TODAY BEST SELLER, *SUCCESS MINDSETS*

Lead2Flourish is the book I wish my leaders had read and practiced when I was pursuing my career in corporate and government. It's a personal and professional growth plan that can be utilized at any stage of one's career. Growth requires intentional actions and a positive environment. This is exactly what makes *Lead2Flourish* so unique and beneficial. Dr. Deana demonstrates that flourishing is a process, not a destination. You must be willing to set your own course and then courageously do it, step by step. If you are serious about being a leader, then this is the book for you. With these tools, we all can become that leader to follow.

—**DIANE BLAKE, Esq.**, LEADERSHIP DEVELOPMENT SPECIALIST AND COMMERCIAL REAL ESTATE INVESTOR

I thoroughly enjoyed reading this book, loved the stories and how Dr. Deana brings herself into the book by sharing mistakes she's made, and lessons learned in her leadership journey. Purposefully reflective and decidedly practical, *Lead2Flourish* is like having your executive coach trained in positive psychology.

—MARGARET H. GREENBERG, MAPP, PCC, CO-AUTHOR OF *THE BUSINESS OF RACE AND PROFIT FROM THE POSITIVE: PROVEN LEADERSHIP*

Lead2Flourish is an essential resource for leaders seeking to identify and overcome the behaviors that are standing in the way of progress and growth. Dr. Deana provides actionable advice and tools that can be applied to your personal and professional life, including your health and wellness.

—PHILIP OVADIA, MD, CARDIOTHORACIC SURGEON AND AUTHOR OF *STAY OFF MY OPERATING TABLE*

Dr. Deana has unlocked the steps leaders need to embody wellbeing and take to be present in a way that inspires and encourages others to bring their best selves to work. Her four stages are easy to follow. The leaders then become models for others to embody a powerful, inspiring presence, breathing life into their organizations. The stories and case studies shared bring the concepts to life. *Lead2Flourish* is a must-read for executives across all industries.

—DR. MARCIA REYNOLDS, AUTHOR OF THE INTERNATIONAL BEST-SELLERS, *COACH THE PERSON, NOT THE PROBLEM* AND *THE DISCOMFORT ZONE: HOW LEADERS TURN DIFFICULT CONVERSATIONS INTO BREAKTHROUGHS*

I've read a lot of leadership books over the last 35 years, and I really like *Lead2Flourish*. Fully researched and documented, *Lead2Flourish* is a broad and essential read on executive behavioral triggers and how it affects your growth and wellbeing. Dr. Deana not only shows a practical and easy-to-understand guide to how and why behavior triggers develop but a real-world intervention plan as well. Whatever your leadership level, *Lead2Flourish* will improve your performance by identifying and eliminating the mental obstacles slowing you down. Ordering copies to grow with my leadership team.

—PETE BOWEN, FORMER ASSISTANT PROFESSOR OF LEADERSHIP AND ETHICS AND AUTHOR OF *ON LEADERSHIP: WHAT'S BROKEN IN OUR SOCIETY AND HOW WE FIX IT*

Executive wellbeing is highly relevant for leadership effectiveness and performance today. Dr. Deana's book, *Lead2Flourish* gives executives the research, the case studies, the lessons, and the process to forgo ego-behavioral patterns and transform themselves, their teams, and their organizations.

—EMILIYA ZHIVOTOVSKAYA, MAPP, MCC, CEO & FOUNDER OF THE FLOURISHING CENTER

Dr. Deana's *Lead2Flourish* science-based blueprint for sustainable behavior change is a must-read to help every leader realize their potential and help their teams do the same. Her simple steps for recognizing unhealthy leadership patterns, renovating destructive behaviors, rebuilding strengths-led habits, and recharging wellbeing ensure this book is full of practical tips every leader can apply.

—**MICHELLE MCQUAID, PH.D., WELLBEING RESEARCHER & FOUNDER OF THE LEADER'S LAB, AUTHOR OF** *YOUR CHANGE BLUEPRINT* **AND** *YOUR STRENGTHS BLUEPRINT*

Lead2Flourish will give you a good dose of personal and professional development in one. With good science and practical examples that will inspire you, Dr. Deana will help you define the root cause of your ego-driven behaviors and renovate your life all in one.

—**LOUIS J. ALLORO, M.ED, MAPP, SENIOR FELLOW, CENTER FOR THE ADVANCEMENT OF WELLBEING**

Lead2Flourish is quite realistic and somewhat reminds me of what I've experienced in business and life. This book is an invaluable cutting-edge resource for helping with the challenges leaders are facing today.

—**THOMAS DONCASTER, CEO of DONCASTER INSURANCE AND FINANCIAL SERVICES**

LEAD 2
FLOURISH

LEAD 2 FLOURISH

An Executive's Guide To Handle
Pressure, Prevent Anxiety, and Lead
From Your Highest Self

Deana Murphy, PhD, CAPP

This publication is designed to provide accurate and authoritative information regarding the subject matter covered. The author and publisher specifically disclaim all liability arising directly or indirectly from the use of any information contained in this book. If legal advice or other expert assistance is required, the services of competent professionals should be sought.

The conversations in this book are based on the author's recollection, though they are not intended to represent word-for-word transcripts. Rather, the author has retold them in a way that communicates the meaning of what was said. In the author's humble opinion, the essence of the dialogue is accurate in all instances.

Copyright @2022 by Deana Murphy
All rights reserved.
No part of this book may be reproduced, stored in a retrieval system, or transmitted by any means electronic, mechanical, photocopying, recording, or otherwise without written permission from the copyright holder, except in the case of brief quotations embodied in critical articles or reviews.

Ordering Information
Quantity sales. Special discounts are available on quantity purchases by corporations, associations, and others. For details, contact Deana@DrDeana.com

Library of Congress Cataloging-in-Publication Data
Names: Murphy, Deana, author
Title: Lead2Flourish: an executive's guide to handle pressure, prevent anxiety, and lead from your highest self / by Deana Murphy.
Identifiers: LCCN 2022916894 | ISBN: 978-0-9864015-2-7 (hardcover) | ISBN: 978-0-9864015-4-1 (paperback) | ISBN: 978-0-9864015-3-4 (audio)

Cover Design by: Taofeek Abdulqoyum
Text Design and Production: Abdul Moiz and Decision Books
Managing Editors: Daniel DeCillis, Hayley Sherman, & Liz Saucedo

To Isaiah and Joshua

*May you and your generation be the leaders
who Lead2Flourish from a foundation of wellbeing.*

I WANT TO HEAR FROM YOU

Please share your feedback on Lead2Flourish with other readers. Please write an honest review of this book at your favorite online bookshop.

★   ★   ★   ★   ★

CONTENTS

---

1   **CHAPTER 1**
       THE ESSENCE TO FLOURISH

       1   Introduction
       4   Moving From Obliviousness to Awareness
       6   The Quagmire Drama
       7   The Cognitive Effect
       10   Why I Wrote This Book

13   **CHAPTER 2**
       LEAD2FLOURISH

       13   Influence Capability
       14   Flourish
       15   Lead2Flourish
       16   Allow Me to Teach You
       18   The R4 Blueprint
       19   Getting the Most Out of This Book

STAGE 1: RECOGNIZING

23   **CHAPTER 3**
       UNCONSCIOUS GAPS & RECOGNIZING ROOT CAUSES

       23   Three Intimate Connections
       24   How Do We Get This Way?
       26   Our Worldview
       27   Our People View
       28   Our Self-View
       29   Adverse Childhood Experiences (ACEs)
       31   Lead2Flourish Keys
       32   Questions for Reflection
       32   Designing a Lead2Flourish Plan – Recognizing Root Causes

33 CHAPTER 4
RECOGNIZING THE TRAPS & THE LIABILITIES

- 33 Stuck In Thoughts
- 34 Recognizing Unhelpful Thought Patterns
- 38 Your Childhood May Have Some Clues
- 38 My Theory Confirmed
- 39 Six Principles Of Recognizing And Undoing Ego-Driven Behavior Patterns
- 43 Lead2Flourish Keys
- 43 Questions for Reflection
- 44 Designing a Lead2Flourish Plan – Recognizing the Traps and Liabilities

45 CHAPTER 5
MYTHS & MISINFORMATION: RECOGNIZING THE DAMAGES

- 45 PANDORA'S BOX OF MYTHS
- 46 BEHAVIOR MYTH #1: OVERTHINKING IS PROBLEM-SOLVING
  - 46 Getting Out of Your Head
  - 47 Meet Paul
  - 49 Meet Gina
  - 50 Overthinking (Ruminating) Concerns
  - 51 Negativity Bias Concerns
  - 51 How?
  - 52 Five Principles Of Excavating The Overthinking Mindset
  - 55 Lead2Flourish Keys
  - 56 Questions for Reflection
  - 56 Designing a Lead2Flourish Plan – The Costs of Overthinking

- 57 BEHAVIOR MYTH #2: MULTITASKING IS TIME MANAGEMENT
  - 57 Ego-Driven Performance
  - 57 Getting to the Brain of Task-switching Behavior
  - 59 Six Principles Of Undoing Task-Switching Behavior
  - 62 Lead2Flourish Keys
  - 62 Questions for Reflection
  - 63 Designing a Lead2Flourish Plan – Undoing the Multitasking Behavior

- 64 BEHAVIOR MYTH #3: FEEDBACK IS CRITICISM
  - 64 Be Like Liz
  - 65 The Breakfast of Champions
  - 65 So Why the Feedback Phobia?
  - 67 How to Recognize Feedback Phobia Behaviors
  - 68 Three Principles Of Undoing Feedback Phobias
  - 70 Lead2Flourish Keys
  - 71 Questions for Reflection
  - 71 Designing a Lead2Flourish Plan – Challenging the Feedback Myth

71 BEHAVIOR MYTH #4: WORK AND LIFE MUST BALANCE

  72 One Life, No Tradeoffs
  72 Meet Natalie
  73 Where Did Work-Life Balance Come From?
  73 Unraveling the Myth
  74 No On and Off Switch
  76 Six Principles Of Integrating Work And Life
  79 Lead2Flourish Keys
  80 Questions for Reflection
  80 Designing a Lead2Flourish Plan – Undoing Work-Life Balance Behavior

STAGE 2: RENOVATING

83 **CHAPTER 6**
  RENOVATING TO REALIZE VALUES: THE GUIDING FOUNDATION

  83 Personal Journey to Realizing Values
  85 Why Renovate to Realize Values
  85 We Are the Behaviors Others See
  86 Answer These Questions
  87 Five Principles Of Value-Driven Behavior
  90 Questions for Reflection – Realizing Values
  91 Lead2Flourish Keys
  92 Designing a Lead2Flourish Plan – Renovating to Realize Values

93 **CHAPTER 7**
  RENOVATING TO REALIZE VISION: WHAT YOU EXPECT TO SEE

  93 The Man in the Park
  94 To See or Not to See
  95 Start With Why
  96 Why We Struggle With "Why"
  97 Limited Options
  97 Limited Resources
  97 Limited Reality
  98 Renovating to Realizing Vision
  98 Vision Requires Purposeful, Driven Behavior
  99 Realizing Purposeful Behavior With Visualization
  100 Two Principles Of Realizing Your Personal Vision
  102 Lead2Flourish Keys
  103 Questions for Reflection
  103 Designing a Lead2Flourish Plan – Renovating to Realize Vision

105 **CHAPTER 8**
  RENOVATING TO REALIZE VOICE: APPRECIATING YOUR BRAND

  105 We've Been Guilty of This
  106 The Leader's Voice

107 Why Renovate to Realize Voice
108 Not Only Women
109 Tearing Down the Myths
112 Five Principles Of Renovating To Realize Voice
115 Lead2Flourish Keys
116 Questions for Reflection
116 Designing a Lead2Flourish Plan – Renovating to Realize Voice

STAGE 3: REBUILDING

121 **CHAPTER 9**
REBUILDING WITH SIGNATURE STRENGTHS: STRENGTH-CENTERED LEADERSHIP

121 Faulty or Unfaulty
122 The Science
123 Signature Strengths Explained
123 Rebuilding Bold Leadership
126 Three Principles Of Rebuilding With Signature Strengths
128 What Follows After Knowing Your Strengths?
128 Lead2Flourish Keys
129 Questions for Reflection
129 Designing a Lead2Flourish Plan – Rebuilding With Signature Strengths

131 **CHAPTER 10**
REBUILDING WITH EMOTIONAL RESILIENCE: ENERGIZED LEADERSHIP

131 Keeping the Sails Steady
133 Responding to Your Pain
134 Opening to Emotional Resilience
135 Rebuilding With Emotional Resilience
136 Six Principles Of Rebuilding With Emotional Resilience
140 Lead2Flourish Keys
140 Questions for Reflection
141 Designing a Lead2Flourish Plan – Rebuilding With Emotional Resilience

143 **CHAPTER 11**
REBUILDING WITH SMART HABITS: EFFICIENT LEADERSHIP

143 Vehicle of a Plan
144 Build Smart Habits. Achieve SMART Goals
145 Habit Research
145 Transferring This Thinking to the Workplace
146 What I Know Now
147 Four Principles Of Rebuilding With Smart Habits
149 Lead2Flourish Keys
150 Questions for Reflection
150 Designing a Lead2Flourish Plan: Rebuilding With Smart Habits

STAGE 4: RECHARGING

153 CHAPTER 12
RECHARGING THE BUSINESS OF WELLBEING:
CONSCIOUS LEADERSHIP

- 153 A Positive Posture
- 155 Discovering Performance Wellbeing
- 158 The Sustaining Tool for Recharging the Business of Wellbeing
- 158 Six Supporting Vitality Behaviors Of Recharging The Business Of Wellbeing
- 168 Lead2Flourish Keys
- 169 Questions for Reflection
- 169 Designing a Lead2Flourish Plan – Recharging the Business of Wellbeing

171 CHAPTER 13
RECHARGING WITH GRATITUDE: SUPPORTIVE LEADERSHIP

- 171 The Remarkable Mr. Mulley
- 173 The Most Attractive Leadership Accessory
- 175 Six Gratitude Behavior Shifts
- 177 Five Principles Of Recharging With Gratitude
- 180 Something to Consider Going Forward
- 180 Lead2Flourish Keys
- 181 Questions for Reflection
- 181 Designing a Lead2Flourish Plan – Recharging with Gratitude

183 FINAL THOUGHTS
187 ACKNOWLEDGMENTS
189 NOTES
195 ABOUT DR. DEANA

LIST OF DIAGRAMS & CHARTS
___

8   "REACTIVE ORIENTED BEHAVIORS"
9   "THE FIGHTING-EGO"
23   "THE THREE INTIMATE CONNECTIONS"
25   "INNATE VS. LEARNED BEHAVIORS"
48   "OVERTHINKING COSTS"
76   "ZEST ZAPPERS"
77   "ENERGY BUILDING"
95   "GOLDEN CIRCLE"
147   "HABIT LOOP"

CHAPTER 1

THE ESSENCE TO FLOURISH

Introduction

You've already heard a plethora of ways to lead. You've attended the leadership development conferences and read the books. You've seen the one-size-fits-all training initiatives. You already know what it takes to be a good leader. And to fuel your drive, you've listened to many motivational speakers. But none of these methods have addressed the root causes of why you lead and behave the way you do or how to get what you want out of life.

More than ever, leaders are facing pressure, fear, and interpersonal issues, leaving a deficit in leadership. Your greatest potential isn't centered on new skills or how-to tips. It's in growing your ability to bring your highest self to every moment, challenge, and relationship. It may feel like the outside world is causing this pressure, but it's your inner ego that's aggressively engaged.

In this book, I'll give you the tools to finetune your thinking and behavior, defy your ego derailers, and lead from a foundation of wellbeing, to operate life from a higher level. This is why you must explore leadership as a personal internal action and create a setting that inspires others to grow and give their best.

My professional roots began with over two decades of service in corporate leadership with companies like Chase and Citigroup. After that, I spent over ten years in the teaching and consulting space, guiding clients both nationally and internationally on personal and professional development, strategy, performance wellbeing, and flourishing. I'm also an architectural interior designer. I'd like to begin our journey together with a story about architectural design that explains what can happen when you demonstrate the essence to flourish.

It was 1929. Oblivious to the impending Great Depression, a group of architectural designers banded together behind the idea of erecting the world's tallest building in Manhattan to eclipse the nearby Chrysler Building owned by their competitor. The site at Fifth Avenue, between 33rd and 34th Streets, had previously been occupied by the Waldorf-Astoria Hotel. They tore the hotel down to build a new symbol of sky-high American "corporate power"—the Empire State Building. According to historians, the contracts with architects Shreve, Lamb, and Harmon Associates were signed in September 1929. The lead architect of the project, William F. Lamb, completed the drawings within two weeks.[1]

About 3,400 construction workers, many of them immigrants from Europe, as well as hundreds of fearless Mohawk Indian ironworkers, came together to build Lamb's design. By employing innovative construction methods and techniques, Lamb inspired the workers to grow and give their best and the framework rose 4 ½ floors a week. Concerned about suicide attempts, Lamb decided to devise measures to prevent people from jumping. The Empire State Building, "the world's tallest building," was completed on time and under budget. Lamb wasn't power-driven, combative, or judgmental and took

CHAPTER 1: The Essence To Flourish

responsibility whenever adjustments were needed.² His sixteenth plan resulted in the building that is still considered one of New York's greatest landmarks.

Lamb's leadership competencies demonstrated new levels of trust, transparency, and collaboration. His personable approach and sociable behaviors made a creative working environment for a diverse staff in which he was able to personally make behavioral corrections where needed. Lamb's production management-based approach to design and construction, seen as an anomaly to traditional practices, played a crucial role in the successful completion of the project.³

Leaders today stand in the equivalent of that 1929 intensely competitive arena on Fifth Avenue in New York. They're operating on autopilot for the sake of attaining corporate power. Department silos and competition are rampant within their companies. Egos are running things. Leaders are unconsciously derailed at the expense of their wellbeing and performance. As an executive leader, you need to understand how you set the tone for the rest of your team, as Lamb did. You need to know how to open the door to new levels of trust, transparency, and collaboration, as with Lamb. You need to exhibit sociable behavior to your diverse staff. You need to know how to make necessary adjustments and change unproductive behaviors. You need to know when to shift your management approach, which plays a crucial role in creating strategic advantages and sustainable business success.

If you want to hone good behavioral competencies, you need to be willing to get uncomfortable to modify your approach. Then, as with Lamb, your management style will be recognized and welcomed as the necessary anomaly to traditional leadership practices.

There are approximately four million visitors to the Empire State Building each year, and researchers at Cornell University concluded in 2011 that the Empire State Building is the most photographed building in the world. As of 2021, the Empire State Building is the fourth-tallest building in New York City and the sixth-tallest building in the United States—because of William F.

Lamb's leadership under uncertain and challenging conditions and the right behavioral competencies, as his best self, to do his best work and modeled this capacity to others.[4]

Lamb's wife told architectural historian Anthony W. Robins, "He [Lamb] knew when it was supposed to be finished there'd be a great to-do . . . and he planned, very deliberately, that we would go abroad that same day [of the building's opening]. And Bill [Lamb] was in a state of absolute delight. The job was done, and well done, and he said, 'Isn't this marvelous? We don't have to listen to all these speeches!' He was so happy."[5] From this story, we can see a leader with unpretentious behavioral skills who congruently gathered a multifaceted, multicultural group of people. He created a context that inspired others to grow and give their best, even while working during a depression, toward a common shared vision. And through all of it, he kept his foot firmly on his ego.

What William F. Lamb demonstrated—from the conception to drawings, to construction to the opening—of that Fifth Avenue colossal in New York City was his essence to flourish. Constantly stretching himself and staying in tune with the world around him, he led the project's construction design with self-awareness, accountability, agility, integrity, and authenticity.

This book addresses how executives today can do the same for their companies. With awareness, the right behavioral competencies, and personal mastery, you can undo unconscious behavior triggers that bring about pressure and anxiety.

Moving From Obliviousness to Awareness

To begin the process of design and construction, first, you need to know the details of what and whom you're working with. You must take a closer look to determine the elements or features that will impact the finished product. Much the same way, an executive's success hangs on knowing and trusting whom you're working with. But the key element to trusting others is knowing and trusting yourself, including knowing how your unconscious,

CHAPTER 1: The Essence To Flourish

unhelpful behaviors and habits impact team dynamics and the organization's bottom line. You may be thinking, "I don't have unconscious, unhelpful behaviors," or, of course, "I know my behaviors." But you'd be surprised by how many leaders, regardless of how long they've been in a leadership role, aren't conscious of their strengths, weaknesses, behaviors, and presence. What they're primarily unaware of are the hidden trigger sources and the impact these behavior tendencies have on others.

Early in my corporate career, I worked alongside high-net-worth real estate executives at one of the largest financial institutions in New York City. Eager to learn and grow within the industry, I saw that the element of inspiration needed in a demanding environment fell short. Despite possessing vast knowledge, the leadership performances showed certain counterproductive aspects that had built up over the years. Plans didn't work out as people thought, and leadership tended not to manifest their vision. This limited both their potential and the potential of the workers. There were power struggles, office politics, offensive behavior patterns, and department silos. The subtle complaining, blaming, excuses, and attention-grabbing idioms weren't unusual or rare. On the surface, it appeared to be entrenched in the DNA. Behavioral issues like these still exist today.

Though behavioral patterns are generally overlooked, they largely define us. There's a lot of truth in the proverb: hindsight is twenty-twenty. It's easy to see the right thing to do or understand something after it's already happened. When you can evaluate yourself and your performance objectively and accurately, it prepares you for both personal and business success. To do this, you must recognize and master your behavior patterns as a whole person, not solely as an executive of a company. Why do so many skillful, competent, and talented leaders flounder in their executions or lose respect and engagement of their people? In hindsight, the answers are clear.

Frustrations sabotage hope and joy, which affects engagement. And yet this is often the accepted culture.

In fact, a Gallup study shows the percentage of actively disengaged employees in the US through June 2021 is 15%. Actively disengaged employees report miserable work experiences and are generally poorly managed.[6] But a more thought-provoking study from the international HR consultants Willis Towers Watson shows that while many people are keen to contribute more at work, the behavior of their managers and the culture of their organizations are actively discouraging them from doing so. Most participants indicated that their supervisors put obstacles in their path. The study, the largest of its kind, was carried out among more than 85,000 people working for large and midsize companies in sixteen countries on four continents.[7]

While these destructive behavior patterns may appear obvious, they're mostly done unconsciously. At first, you may not even notice that you're doing it. But when these habits consistently undermine your efforts, they can be considered a form of psychological self-harm, not to mention the possible harm caused to others. They can seriously damage your confidence and reputation. Here's how I was caught up in this quagmire and overcame it.

The Quagmire Drama

It wasn't uncommon for John, our division head, to have impromptu meetings. When he called me to his office, I went prepared with a pen and pad. Before I could sit down and without justification, he insinuated I'd neglected to follow up on a situation with one of my property owners, Mr. Miller. He then handed me his phone. Guess who was on the line: Mr. Miller. Embarrassed and appalled by the episode, I took the receiver and spoke with Mr. Miller, hoping to get an understanding of the issue. In my mind, it was a baseless mistake. And as it turned out, I hadn't neglected anything. Mr. Miller had what he needed but was merely looking for some follow-up clarification.

Before getting the facts, John was obliviously unaware that he'd shifted from a *'creative'* orientation to a *'reactive'* orientation. He surrendered to his often-seen, bull-headed, egotistical survival mechanism. He saw his ego as his

CHAPTER 1: The Essence To Flourish

strength often demonstrated by impatience and an insensitive way of holding people accountable. John wasn't aware, and neither did he understand, that he had a damaging behavior problem. Later I learned that, in a nasty attempt to undermine me, the entire drama was orchestrated by one of my managing colleagues who had initially received Mr. Miller's call. Instead of referring Mr. Miller directly to me, she sent the call to John, knowing in advance the way he impulsively reacted in situations like these.

It's not uncommon for leaders to jump to conclusions before they obtain the facts. As for my colleague's role, it's sad that some leaders may enjoy stirring up drama. Although her childish behavior appeared deliberate, perhaps there were past experiences that triggered her conduct. I very much doubt that she was innocently unaware of the potential consequences that would follow. This is a grave mistake for any leader. Encouraging or participating in this kind of behavior can put you in a downward spiral, making the situation continuously worse. It can also create a rift among the workforce. You'll never be content placing blame or complaining about someone else. You'll only ruin your essence to flourish.

The Cognitive Effect

The brain is skilled at creating strong feelings and self-justifications. That's what happened to John. He unconsciously feared that my alleged mistake would reflect poorly on him. When he perceived that his reputation was threatened, he was triggered to react. Lashing out was one of his ways of surviving. Because these tendencies are so entrenched, they can happen spontaneously in the presence of stress, pressure, fear, or loss. You may be viewed as intelligent, highly competent, and cool, but harmful behaviors will negatively impact your colleagues and the company culture and are detrimental to effective management.

The reality is that 95% of your thinking, feeling, believing, and actions are driven by your unconscious automatic processing. What drives much of that unconscious automatic processing? Your mindset. Your mindset is the mental funnel that fuels your thinking, learning, and behavior. Consequently, it also fuels the effectiveness of your leadership, your success, and the degree to which your organization is agile. Whether or not you are conscious of your mindset activity, it dictates the direction of your life.

Below are some common examples of reactive-oriented behavior. Can you recognize any of them?

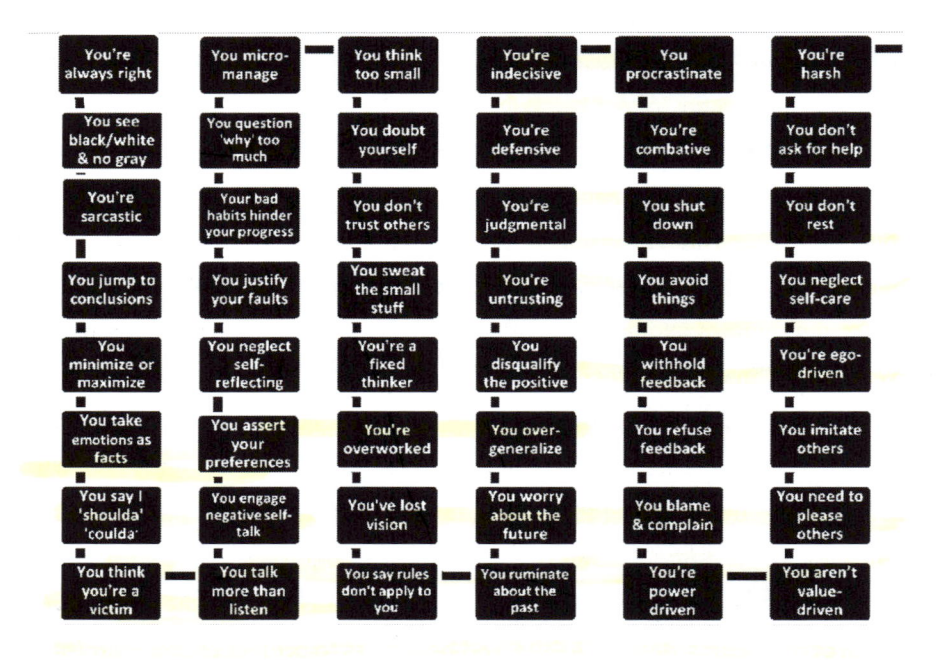

You're always right	You micro-manage	You think too small	You're indecisive	You procrastinate	You're harsh
You see black/white & no gray	You question 'why' too much	You doubt yourself	You're defensive	You're combative	You don't ask for help
You're sarcastic	Your bad habits hinder your progress	You don't trust others	You're judgmental	You shut down	You don't rest
You jump to conclusions	You justify your faults	You sweat the small stuff	You're untrusting	You avoid things	You neglect self-care
You minimize or maximize	You neglect self-reflecting	You're a fixed thinker	You disqualify the positive	You withhold feedback	You're ego-driven
You take emotions as facts	You assert your preferences	You're overworked	You over-generalize	You refuse feedback	You imitate others
You say I 'shoulda' 'coulda'	You engage negative self-talk	You've lost vision	You worry about the future	You blame & complain	You need to please others
You think you're a victim	You talk more than listen	You say rules don't apply to you	You ruminate about the past	You're power driven	You aren't value-driven

Reactive behaviors like these are like having another mind within your mind. This other mind is your ego, and it prompts an unconscious automatic reaction when threatened and collides with your emotions. For example, believing that your team members disrespect the work you're producing makes you apprehensive about pushing forward with the heartfelt ideas you want to explore. No one has said anything directly to you, but your emotional reasoning becomes suspicious of others' actions. Your ego is threatened. Your unconscious automatic reaction is to not trust them. Defending yourself and

CHAPTER 1: The Essence To Flourish

justifying your work ethic is how you 'fight back' to remain in your comfort zone. All the while, you aren't aware that these dysfunctional behavior patterns are canceling the essence to flourish by leading you directly away from creativity.

At my company, we refer to these dysfunctional behavior patterns as the *fighting-ego syndrome*. The *fighting-ego* looks like this: You're triggered by a belief (ego threat). You react (unhelpful behavior without a conscious choice of how to respond). You defend (guided by believing your reputation might be smeared). You justify (protecting your *fighting-ego* patterns). Can you think of more common examples of reactive-oriented behavior?

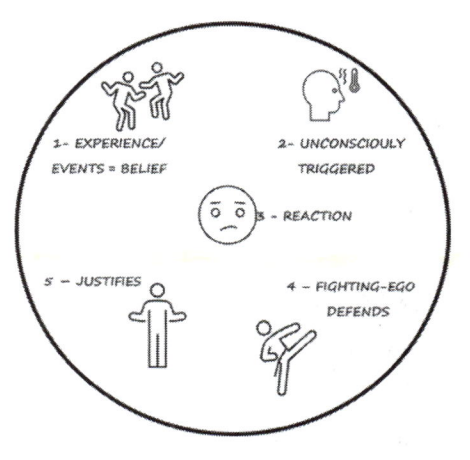

1- EXPERIENCE/ EVENTS = BELIEF
2- UNCONSCIOULY TRIGGERED
3 - REACTION
4 – FIGHTING-EGO DEFENDS
5 – JUSTIFIES

As you can see from the reactive-oriented behavior chart, many automatic reactions may seem like personality traits. They are survival behaviors triggered by overreacting to a threat to the ego. The ego is a part of us that engages in self-justification that has both cognitive and motivational functions. Its main purpose is to develop self-protection mechanisms in the form of our beliefs, desires, habits, and behaviors to protect us from our fears. When our egos are challenged, as John's was, or hurt by others, we are prone to becoming triggered.

It happens to all of us. Our triggers set us off into a tirade of hostile, fearful, angry, or resentful behaviors toward those who pose a threat to our ego's survival. Our subconscious often contains a set of insecurities that stemmed from painful experiences in our childhood. Because our brains are wired to protect us from reliving this pain, it's on hyper-alert to those triggers, which become unconscious ego threats. No worries. This book is your guide to undoing these unconscious patterns so you can develop the essence to flourish in leadership, life, and society and be more empowered to better the future of humanity.

Cognitive-behavioral approaches have been studied extensively and are highly effective at finetuning both thinking and behavior to give you the best positive impact.[8] I believe these approaches will resonate with leaders like you at any organizational level as they water down the usual theories and idealistic views often taken in traditional leadership publications.

My personal view of the leadership industry is colored by my experience with leaders in corporate, consulting, and coaching spaces, where big egos and unrealized fears get in the way of growth. I can personally connect with this. As an only child, I compensated with the need to come out on top of things. My cousins often teased and taunted me when I discussed the wonderful things I wanted to do with my life. Throughout both elementary and high school, my classmates sometimes mocked me with "Who do you think you are?" or "The girl who thinks she's better than us." My ego was sorely bruised because that wasn't how I wanted to be portrayed. I turned inwardly to my self-protective mechanisms, my insecurities, and my doubts.

My sense of insecurity as a child continued to have a great impact on my adult life as a leader. I had a sharp tongue and the need to always be right. While believing these were my strengths, they were unwanted liabilities. I kept quiet when I needed to speak up and spoke up when I needed to keep quiet. There wasn't a safe place to explore my frustrations, making it difficult to align my actions with what I valued and envisioned for my life. I later learned that my wellbeing and performance suffered as a result.

Why I Wrote This Book

My studies in cognitive behavior and applied psychology helped me discover how to liberate myself from unhelpful thinking styles and behaviors and go beyond the ego. My roles as teacher, speaker, and consulting positive psychologist have thrust me into putting practical, positive psychology

CHAPTER 1: The Essence To Flourish

research into action—traveling internationally to support clients. I have witnessed the remarkable breakthroughs that are possible when we're released from the constrictions of our limiting beliefs and unconscious, unproductive behaviors. I've successfully taught many others to improve themselves; now, I want to teach you.

While exploring the science of flourishing, behavior, and wellbeing, I discovered a quote by D. Bender in an employee assistance program (EAP) article, "Trouble at the Top," where he said, "Studies indicate that one in six executives is troubled by personal problems that affect his job performance."[9] In addition, the 2021 Bupa Global Executive Wellbeing Index captured disturbing insights from its poll of high-net-worth individuals and senior executives about their work, home, and health. They surveyed over 1,200 executives based across Europe, North America, the Middle East, and Asia which showed work-related wellbeing has fallen by 45% since the onset of the pandemic. Three-quarters (77%) of the senior executives and high-net-worth individuals surveyed suffered at least one symptom associated with poor mental health in the past year—up from 70% in 2020.[10]

The challenges of this volatile, uncertain, complex, ambiguous (VUCA) world weigh heavily on organizations and their leaders, teams, and people. So, I'm taking what I've learned to those who have a lot to do but with less— executive leaders. Doing a lot with less can wear you down physically, emotionally, psychologically, spiritually, and relationally.

The idea emerged in a visionary phrase during my morning prayer and meditation: *Lead2Flourish*. That's exactly how I saw it: one phrase as one word without spelling out the number two. At first, I thought it was simply a cool slogan. At the time, I honestly had no clue where or how to fit it into my work or if I should. But I felt that it was part of a much bigger picture.

Linking the components of flourishing with the dynamics of leadership in my mind achieves the missing element in the leadership development equation. And there it was. Clearer and clearer, I grasped the intent of

LEAD2FLOURISH

Lead2Flourish—a holistic and comprehensive approach to mainstream leadership development programs with a focus on unconscious behavioral change—transcending your current state to a new level of consciousness. This relates to behavioral intelligence, a skillset used to understand and suppress emotional triggers to execute, at will, helpful behaviors and be effective with people and challenging situations. Then, the concept of behavioral intelligence and human flourishing became my leadership model that supports, sustains, and secures performance wellbeing over time.

In response to these desires, *Lead2Flourish* was created, which I'm excited to introduce to you in this book. Like William F. Lamb's production management-based approach to the construction of the Empire State Building, the *Lead2Flourish* performance-wellbeing approach is my cutting-edge contribution to leadership development.

With pleasure and gratitude, I give you what I've learned to help you undo your unhelpful behavioral tendencies unleashing the essence to flourish that allows you to enjoy more of what you do.

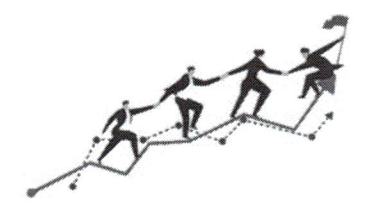

CHAPTER 2

LEAD2FLOURISH

Influence Capability

You probably picked up this book because you have influence or authority over others. That identifies you as a leader, in particular, an executive leader. Do you know why you're in the leadership business? How did you gravitate toward influencing others? Are you leading from your highest self? Are you connected with whom you want to be as a leader? Do you step fully into your leadership role with creativity and courage? Do you lead with a personal vision? What explodes on the inside of you when you think of leading others? Is it fear? Is it anxiety? Is it tension? Is it a success edge? Are you spending time on what matters most? How is the energy among those you lead? Is your ego considered a leadership strength? How well do you work across silos? Your responses to questions like these determine if you lead and flounder or *Lead2Flourish*.

Flourish

"Flourish" is seen in the title of many books, courses, and businesses. "Flourish" occurs thirty-two times in eleven translations of the Bible. Why is it such a popular word? "Flourish" is creating a good, full life that's grounded in wellbeing. "Flourish" is a state we create when we raise resilience, outsmart stress, and elevate engagement with the world and our work. "Flourish" results from pursuing an authentic life as we connect passions with meaningful work and savor our accomplishments through life's twists and turns.

"Flourish," is engaging the behaviors and habits that build the best qualities in life. When we flourish, we expand both the range of what we do and the depth with which we do it. That's what this book will help you do: use your internal resources to expand the range and depth of what you do, achieving external flourishing results.

Human Flourishing—those were the words I'd frequently tossed around in my mind. They were magnetic and inviting in a way that pulled me in with curiosity. My work in this area is sourced from great teachers of philosophy, neuroscience, behavioral science, performance management, and applied psychology. Scholars such as Martin Seligman, Adam Grant, Barbara Fredrickson, Aaron Beck, and many others—collecting their perspectives, principles, and practices to understand what it is to flourish and experience total life wellbeing when faced with high demands, adversity, and uncertainties.

Though each of these scholars may use a different context for looking at human flourishing, most psychologists agree that flourishing goes beyond the notion of unpretentious happiness and wellbeing. It offers a more holistic perspective of the way we live, work, and relate to one another. To move toward flourishing, Organizational Psychologist Adam Grant, one of Wharton's top-rated professors for over seven years, encourages us to focus

CHAPTER 2: LEAD2FLOURISH

on our purpose. Why are we here? How do we inject meaning into our day-to-day work?[1] And I might add, why do we lead? Flourishing concepts like these gave me a strong appetite to explore and discover more, so I could share more with you.

Lead2Flourish

Lead2Flourish is a science-based skillset—a blueprint for sustainable behavioral change. It helps leaders to hone behavioral intelligence and lead from their highest selves, do their best work, and model this capacity to others. This book guides you in the ways to identify, bravely yet uncomfortably, some of the deepest, below-the-surface thoughts, feelings, assumptions, and beliefs to understand who you are as a leader. And primarily, this book addresses the root causes of why you act the way you do.

In fact, McKinsey talked with hundreds of chief executives about the most common mistakes companies make in their leadership development efforts and identified changing behaviors and adjusting mindsets as one of four oversights.[2] It's time to shift the leadership context, regarding the performance and wellbeing subject, to flourishing—taking it from a meager secondary idea to an essential foundation for leadership success. Why?

In leadership training, the focus has mainly been on employee wellness, workplace engagement, diversity, and inclusion. Executive wellbeing has been overlooked. Until we correct the *fighting-ego syndrome*, it will get us more of what we don't want: dysfunctional individuals, families, societies, communities, and organizations.

Over the past twenty-four months, I have explored and studied executive wellbeing and made the behavior-performance connection. And this must be in place at the outset to effectively implement any employee-focused area. Carrying any decision-making role requires the capacity to perform efficiently, expressed by who you are rather than what you do before you can answer both the needs of others and those of the company.

Executives have borne the brunt of both frustrations and floundering because of employee quit rates and vaccine mandates. The COVID debacle has highlighted what was already becoming clear before its emergence: that we don't need ego-driven leaders. The most effective leadership today—at all levels—isn't always about outsmarting the competition, asserting technical expertise, and having all the answers. It's about having the *Lead2Flourish* competence—a state created when you're in control of your behavioral intelligence and can shine in all life domains: your private life, your work, your home, your relationships, your communities, and tying these together instead of hopelessly trying to balance them.

Lead2Flourish also requires a conscious effort to respond to life instead of unconsciously reacting to it. Psychiatrist Viktor Frankl understood the freedom in living by this philosophy, citing in his memoir, *Man's Search for Meaning*, "Between stimulus and response there is a space. In this space is our power to choose our response. In our response lies our growth and our freedom."[3]

Allow Me to Teach You

Based on the definition of human flourishing, I've put together a blueprint to get you to a flourishing place as a leader. In my simple and easy-to-understand way, I'll guide you to become the lead architect in the construction of your inner and outer life. I want to arm you with the knowledge of how to handle pressure and even prevent anxiety, all based on sound and published evidence. You'll learn how to recognize and undo the ego-protected behaviors to drive functional, innovative leadership.

Together, we'll identify the unconscious behavior patterns that get in your way. I'll teach you how to hold a mirror to your life and dig up the root causes of the behavior patterns that hijack your best performance. I'll teach you how to rewire your thinking. As an outcome, you'll make better choices and decisions, you'll perform with poise and confidence, and you'll handle work

CHAPTER 2: LEAD2FLOURISH

more efficiently with more mental energy to weather stressors and manage personal challenges. In other words, you'll get the alignment, wellbeing, and efficiency you need to *Lead2Flourish* and enjoy life more.

In the following pages, you'll meet leaders whom I've worked with in the corporate landscape and in teaching, coaching, and consulting settings. You'll discover how their experiences have shaped their beliefs, values, and behaviors and how these experiences impacted their performance, wellbeing, and capacity to flourish. You'll discover that seemingly innocent behaviors can be unhelpful and how they insidiously hijack personal and professional progress. You'll learn the ways your *fighting-ego* restricts you. You'll learn how to recognize its hidden triggers and unmask the myths with strategies, interventions, exercises, and plans to move forward.

In understanding and undoing how your behavior can be seized by unconscious tendencies, I'll provide simple, actionable tools that:

- Have an existing body of research to support their reliability
- Are evidence-based
- Are sustainably beneficial

I'll present solutions to problems that concern every leader, such as:

- How do I balance the demands placed on me and cultivate smart habits?
- How can I give 100% and have the mental energy to develop a greater impact?
- How do I raise my performance and sustain my wellbeing?

When you have more challenges than resources, your wellbeing dips, along with your capacity to flourish, and vice versa. Following Sonja Lyubomirsky's contention that 40% of one's intentional strategies will differentiate the flourishing from their non-flourishing colleagues,[4] your

LEAD2FLOURISH

responsibility is to consciously put this capacity in your own hands. The *Lead2Flourish* blueprint is a compelling representation of the factors known to guide you to this end. Everything you're going to read in the coming pages creates sustainable changes that I live by every day.

The R4 Blueprint

To meet this need, the four-stage *Lead2Flourish* reconstruction blueprint is my forward-thinking contribution to leadership development, designed to undo the unhelpful, unconscious, ego-protected behaviors (floundering) and then create the path for modeling the change wanted in teams, organizations, and communities (flourishing).

Stage One – *Recognizing*

The conception stage is where we recognize the elements and features that will impact your finished project. Following that practice, we'll start with an evidence-based, nonjudgmental process of recognizing your past unhealthy beliefs, ingrained dysfunctions, survival mechanisms, automatic reactions, and unhelpful behavior patterns that are destructive to performance and wellbeing (Chapters 3 through 5).

Stage Two – *Renovating*

Sometimes we must tear down the old to build the new. We'll renovate dysfunctional, destructive behaviors that interfere with your true essence, expressed in the consistency of your vision, values, and voice, and deconstruct behavior myths that undermine your progress. This design stage helps with aligning ethical decision-making, workplace demands, and cultivating a genuine connection with people and work (Chapters 6 through 8).

Stage Three – *Rebuilding*

After renovating, it's time to rebuild. Just as the structural and mechanical plans must carry the weight of a building's designated activities, we'll rebuild

CHAPTER 2: LEAD2FLOURISH

the often overlooked and unrefined attributes of your core strengths, emotional resilience, and unhelpful habits to equip you to carry the weight of your day-to-day duties, pursuits, and performance (Chapters 9 through 11).

Stage Four – *Recharging*

In this stage, we'll inspect your punch list as a safeguard to keep everything performing smoothly. We'll anchor and strengthen supportive behaviors using intentional self-management practices to recharge wellbeing and performance. We'll help you with getting the needed alignment, efficiency, and genuine earnestness for you to flourish in life and work (Chapters 12 through 13).

Getting the Most Out of This Book

Lead2Flourish research, interventions, and activities are designed for use as a self-guided, at-your-own-pace tool to learn, reflect, take action, and integrate effective conscious behaviors into your life. Do something each day to take you toward flourishing by seeking to recognize, renovate, rebuild, and recharge your inner life for outward success. The process is most effective when you explore the stages in the order presented.

Stop and ponder the reflective questions by simply writing keywords on little sticky notes as reminders or adding them to your reminder app on your smartphone. Find a quiet place where you're undisturbed. You can journal your thoughts about what inspires you as you read. There are a few journaling apps you can download to help. The idea is to do the exercises and act on what you read. You can also weave these exercises into psychological or spiritual activities, such as psychotherapy, meditation, or prayer if you choose. Then you can also mentor and model your productive behaviors to others. The practices and exercises are very simple, so don't make them complicated. Simplicity must never become a lost value. It takes time.

LEAD2FLOURISH

However you decide to get the best out of this book, think about how different your life will be when you have: a flourishing mindset, a flourishing attitude, a flourishing body, a flourishing business, a flourishing career, and a flourishing life. What would it mean to you, to your family, to your existence if this was your experience?

See yourself creating positive and productive experiences for yourself and others. See yourself connecting with whom you want to be as a leader, performing at your best, leading from your highest self, and being the most helpful resource possible for yourself and others. See yourself living to *Lead2Flourish*.

See yourself enjoying life more. Can you see it? Keep sight of it because that's where we're going.

Now you know where we're going, let's get started.

We have work to do.

STAGE 1

RECOGNIZING

The conception stage is where we recognize the elements and features that will impact your finished project. Following that practice, in this stage, we'll start with an evidence-based nonjudgmental process of recognizing your past unhealthy beliefs, ingrained dysfunctions, survival mechanisms, automatic reactions, and unhelpful behavior patterns that are destructive to your performance and wellbeing.

CHAPTER 3

UNCONSCIOUS GAPS & RECOGNIZING ROOT CAUSES

Three Intimate Connections

Unhelpful thoughts have become a "comfortable" part of our mindset. We act on our thoughts. I refer to them as unconscious gaps. Psychologist Aaron T. Beck demonstrated, in his 1960 development of the cognitive model, that one's thoughts and beliefs affect one's behavior and subsequent actions.[1] These factors influence our wellbeing, as illustrated below.

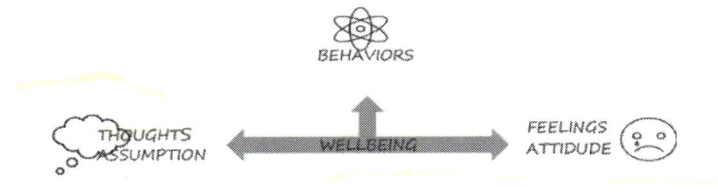

BEHAVIORS

THOUGHTS / ASSUMPTION ⟷ WELLBEING ⟷ FEELINGS / ATTITUDE

To clarify, according to Reuters, Wells Fargo's CEO and President, Charlie Scharf, repeatedly expressed the company's inability to reach its diversity goals over a summer period with the rationale that "there is a very limited pool of Black talent to recruit from."

This behavior exasperated some Black employees. An outbreak of critical comments also flooded the newsfeed on LinkedIn. Scharf's impulsive and inappropriate behavior caused him to later go on record to say, "I apologize for making an insensitive comment reflecting my own unconscious bias."[2]

Because of his ill-thinking and unfavorable attitude (this thought led to a particular harmful feeling/belief), Scharf repeatedly expressed the opinion [thought/assumption/perception] with the rationale [belief] that "there is a very limited pool of Black talent to recruit from" [reaction = behavior = biased]. These beliefs focused his attention on the negative, which unconsciously maneuvered his feelings toward insensitivity and bias. Perceptions play a pivotal role in our wellbeing and how we perform, which is why it's especially important to keep them grounded.

As we'll understand in this chapter, our *fighting-ego* can trigger us to act against our own best interests. This unconscious, automatic reaction can influence our decision-making and our actions, even when we're not aware of it. They slip out when we least expect them to. Dysfunctional practices like these can have a huge boomerang effect on our performance, wellbeing, and influence. Scharf admitted he was triggered by his *behavior bias*, showing that he recognized the behavior; however, he may have been unaware of its source. Once we recognize the root sources and discover the patterns, it's easier to close this gap and work positively toward our goals.

How Do We Get This Way?

Some behaviors are innate, and others are learned. Innate behaviors are inherent and come at birth, while learned behaviors are acquired from experience or the outside environment. Here, I am referring to learned

CHAPTER 3: Unconscious Gaps & Recognizing Root Causes

behaviors. Research shows that a single bad event is stronger than our single strongest good event and can have long-term, harmful consequences. For example, just one case of child abuse or sexual abuse can lead to depression, relationship problems, and re-victimization[3] and have a powerful impact than dozens of happy memories, like birthday parties or trips to the park.

These are usually triggered on a recurring basis. Flip back to the examples listed in Chapter 1 to see what I mean. You hardly notice them until the consequences show up in your work, relationships, and lifestyle. That's why they're considered unconscious behaviors, generally shaped by some hidden event or experience. Note the differences between innate and learned behaviors in the diagram here:

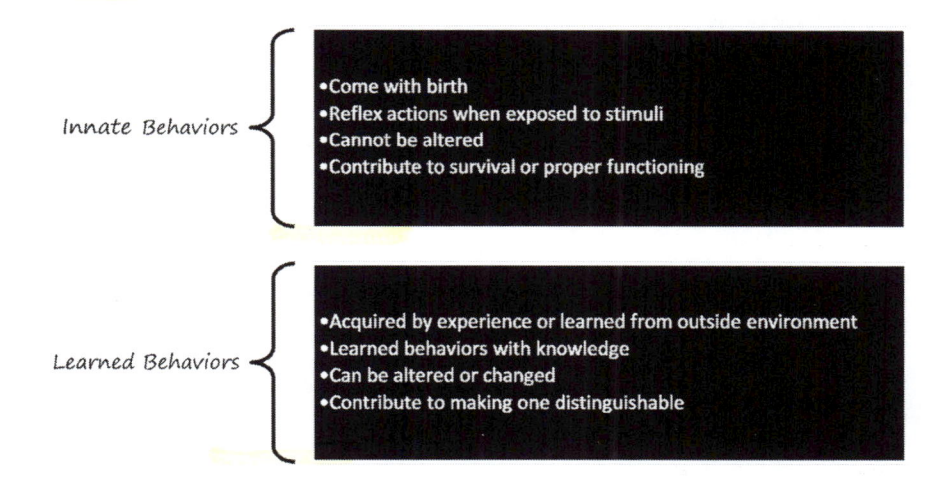

Innate Behaviors
- Come with birth
- Reflex actions when exposed to stimuli
- Cannot be altered
- Contribute to survival or proper functioning

Learned Behaviors
- Acquired by experience or learned from outside environment
- Learned behaviors with knowledge
- Can be altered or changed
- Contribute to making one distinguishable

As people become aware of their unconscious behaviors, or when someone calls them out, typically, they justify them by reacting this way: "That's just the way I am"; "I can't help I was made this way"; "It's part of my personality." The truth is, most behaviors aren't just the way we are; we weren't made this way, nor are they part of our personality. Given that we learned this behavior and developed it over the years, we can learn a different behavior.

Recognizing them and then probing the social component as far back as our childhood for the possible root connections allows us to discover why we think and act a certain way. And by undoing these tendencies, we peel back our natural strengths, talents, and creativity.

I've identified three factors that play a role in fueling unconscious behaviors: *our worldview*, *our people view*, and *our self-view*—all defined by the way we cognitively process and evaluate childhood events.

Our Worldview

The chances are that either you or someone you know resembles my client, Marie, a Vice President of a Fortune 500 financial organization. She spent many years experiencing shame because of an unpredictable and fearful life as the daughter of an alcoholic. Because of her father's lifestyle, she also suffered the experience of a lot of quarreling and conflict during her childhood.

Early on, Marie believed she could erase this family scar by becoming the first to get a college degree. In her mind, Marie had to demonstrate a flawless performance if she was to be successful at managing others. She focused on exceeding expectations at any cost and held her team to the same standards, sometimes far beyond what they could reasonably achieve.

When her team didn't meet these demands, instead of engaging them in the process and approaching the situation effectively, she countered her pent-up frustration with the cold shoulder. Keeping silent, remaining elusive, and avoiding her team caused noticeably emotionally stressful working conditions. Her team became restless and angry and showed low self-esteem. Marie's reactions put an obvious strain on the environment. When the unthinkable happened, and Marie was fired, she blamed everyone but herself.

Or perhaps you can relate to Ben. During his parent's divorce hearing, at age nine, he told the judge he wanted to live with his father. Later, Ben realized he'd made the wrong decision. His father didn't embrace or praise him and

CHAPTER 3: Unconscious Gaps & Recognizing Root Causes

hardly showed loving emotion toward him. Ben desperately missed his mother's nurturing. Having a successful career in a tech firm, he seemed fine before his promotion as the team leader.

But out of nowhere, Ben suddenly became an uncontrolled procrastinator. His decision to keep putting off assignments resulted in losing sight of the bigger picture. To get things moving, he made poor decisions, some of which compromised his values. When things weren't getting done, Ben blamed his team.

This pattern of behavior created an environment of mistrust and team controversy, causing serious structure and accountability issues within his department.

Both Marie and Ben harbored a cynical worldview. The father's image of protection and safety was nonexistent in their world. For them, love and approval were something to be earned, not given, which led to Marie's perfectionist and Ben's procrastinating workplace behavior.

Our People View

Jerry grew up a military brat. Because his father was frequently deployed to different stations, taking the family with him, Jerry had a host of private tutors along the way. He was commonly praised for his work. After a lifetime of praise, not only did he become addicted, but he'd also come to expect it.

Consequently, his desire for praise continued to influence his behavior as director of a data services company. He attended a management meeting in hopes of collaborating with a colleague. Jerry mostly needed to be surrounded by people who encouraged his development and growth. Instead, he left the meeting irritated and angry.

Soon after, he became confrontational and arrogant. He was later overheard complaining about not being appreciated, jabbering about his superiority, and questioning the qualifications of his colleagues. This hit the rumor mill. But Jerry wasn't at all embarrassed by the rumor. He couldn't see why it was a big deal. Remember, he was the army brat.

On the day of that management meeting, in his briefcase, Jerry packed his high self-value and rational egotism and brought them with him to work. Others were a mere backdrop to the world around him. Jerry's narcissistic workplace behaviors created a stressful and tense environment. As a result, his colleagues no longer wanted to work with him. A couple of his colleagues asked to be transferred to a different department.

Our Self-View

Travis is a classic Type A, multi-tasker, device-carrying business analyst for a pharmaceutical company. After both parents died at a young age, he lived with his aunt and uncle, who were much older than his parents. They never had children of their own. Giving him a place to stay and providing food and clothing was their way of showing him love. But Travis still lived with a great sense of loss. His *fighting-ego* desperately wanted more.

To fill this void, in high school, Travis identified with high achievement and had an unshakeable faith in himself. His life became about pushing to change in a more confident direction. Being productive is generally described as providing a large number of positive results. But sometimes, we take it too far and become addicted to busyness, as Travis did. His work spilled over into nights, weekends, vacations, and family celebrations. Emails were sent and received at any hour, day or night. Texting late at night became the norm. And like any other addiction, the good feeling numbed the negative consequences of his actions.

Because of his high-level self-worth and favorable opinion of himself, his unconscious, automatic reaction was to go to any length to prove that he was an achiever. But there was a downside. Travis was often driven by his unconscious desire to be liked. His hurt ego became fueled by a sense of

CHAPTER 3: Unconscious Gaps & Recognizing Root Causes

pressure and anxiety about too much to do and too little time. The cost of these patterns caused him severe exhaustion. Eventually, he called in sick regularly.

Adverse Childhood Experiences (ACEs)

In each of these cases, outwardly successful people manifested unconscious, self-destructive behaviors rooted in their childhood experiences. In fact, studies on Adverse Childhood Experiences (ACEs) have shown that stressful childhood experiences are also linked to various negative social consequences and an increased risk of behavioral and psychological problems, as well as other chronic health conditions.[4]

According to the Texas Institute for Child and Family Wellbeing, the fact that trauma impacts motivation and behavior is not new or surprising to clinicians. "Most of us know when there is something deeper driving a client's behaviors even when it is not articulated."[5]

Award-winning science journalist Donna Jackson Nakazawa explains it in her book, *Childhood Disrupted: How Your Biography Becomes Your Biology, and How You Can Heal*: "When we're thrust over and over again into stress-inducing situations during childhood or adolescence, our physiological stress response shifts into overdrive, and we lose the ability to respond appropriately and effectively to future stressors—ten, twenty, even thirty, years later."

As children, our brain is hard at work, trying to make sense of the world around us. Kids who come into adolescence with a history of adversity and lack the presence of a consistent, loving adult to help them through it may become more likely to develop mood disorders or have poor executive functioning and decision-making skills."

In fact, every time we react to a report, criticize someone's opinion, vent about another department, or judge others who outperform us, we extend a context of mood disorders and unconscious behaviors.[6] Poor performance, the inability to flourish in the company, and the inability to adapt to adversity can be the consequence.

Marie, Ben, Jerry, and Travis were sufferers of Adverse Childhood Experiences (ACEs). As children, it is scary for us when we experience fear, separation, pain, and loss. Our natural survival mechanism wants to avoid them in the future. Marie's, Ben's, Jerry's, and Travis' survival behaviors as children continued to impact them into adulthood as leaders. Let's examine their survival instincts a little closer.

Marie's survival instinct to avoid feeling unloved kept her from letting down her guard and sharing ideas with her team. Fears and anxiety came with the price of losing common sense and level-headedness. Marie believed early on that to be loved and respected, not rejected, meant being a perfectionist. This became her survival behavior when placed in an uncomfortable or challenging situation.

Ben wanted to succeed as a team leader and feared that if he continued making quick decisions, it would reflect poorly on his competence. His survival instinct to procrastinate limited his potential and the potential of the company. So, blaming others became an unconscious attempt to avoid being judged.

After working with Marie and Ben, they recognized their worldview of having to earn love and approval was the trigger behind the *fighting-ego* behaviors. By recognizing their limiting patterns, Marie and Ben worked to make headway toward behavioral intelligence and in clarifying goals so they could commit their energies and effort in the right direction and live more purposefully.

Jerry couldn't relate to others around him because he focused only on himself. He lacked awareness of the importance of others. His need to be important and revered was driven by fear of being rejected by his peers. Jerry realized how many relationships he'd lost because of his behavior and how that limited his performance. After we worked together, Jerry focused on how

CHAPTER 3: Unconscious Gaps & Recognizing Root Causes

he wanted to behave rather than how he wanted to be seen, which resulted in treating others with respect and concern.

Travis' unconscious fear of underperforming was limiting his productivity. His work addiction created a desire to move on from project to project due to a fear that if he wasn't working, he was inefficient and wasting time. As we worked on his understanding of this self-limiting behavior pattern, he was able to realign his objectives.

These leaders learned how to process their past to avoid reliving their pains, find intrinsic motivation in the face of pressure and adversity, and reconnect with their inspiration to make a larger difference.

What about you? This is a good place to discover your *Flourishing IQ* and current stage of wellbeing by taking a *Lead2Flourish* assessment at www.DrDeana.com/assessment.

Lead2Flourish Keys

1. Part of the *Lead2Flourish* design involves recognizing our survival instincts—the thoughts and beliefs we developed as children that show up in adulthood and hinder or limit our progress.
2. What we think, how we feel, and how we behave are all closely connected, and all of these factors have a decisive influence on our wellbeing.
3. The *fighting-ego* can trigger us to act against our own best interests.
4. Research shows that a single bad event is stronger than our single strongest good event and can have long-term harmful consequences.
5. Our worldview, our people's view, and our self-view are three factors that play a role in fueling unconscious behaviors and are defined by the way childhood events are cognitively processed and evaluated.

6. Stressful childhood experiences are also linked to various negative social consequences and an increased risk of behavioral and psychological problems, as well as other chronic health conditions.

Questions for Reflection

1. Ask yourself how your past experiences might be affecting your psychological and physiological wellbeing. This matters because we are less effective and most disruptive when our unconscious behaviors are triggered.
2. What is your worldview, people's view, and/or self-view, and how might these affect your thinking, beliefs, and actions?

Designing a Lead2Flourish Plan – Recognizing Root Causes

Reflecting on what you've learned in this chapter, practice thinking about where you may have unconscious gaps. The goal is to recognize how protecting your ego has played into your personal and professional behaviors and decisions. No one will see this but you. So put your ego on pause and be honest with yourself.

1. Areas where I likely have unconscious gaps: (example: areas where potentials are limited)
2. I will commit to: (example: committing to intentionally being more aware of . . .)
3. My likely *fighting-ego* hurdles are:
4. My timeline:

CHAPTER 4

RECOGNIZING THE TRAPS & THE LIABILITIES

Stuck In Thoughts

Philosopher Marcus Aurelius once said, "Our life is what our thoughts make it." Our thought processes, emotions, and reasons for acting are an important part of making better decisions. What if I told you that your thoughts could trap you, alter your behavior and decisions, and, as a result, control your life?

What we believe now is a by-product of what we've thought about—influenced by our culture and other people. Beliefs, then, are a collection of continual thoughts that have shaped themselves into a conviction. These are areas where we get stuck. We become trapped in different patterns and behaviors we may not even know we are falling into. These patterns not only impact management and team dynamics but also our performance, wellbeing, and ability to flourish.

Recognizing Unhelpful Thought Patterns

Here's a design illustration that highlights the direction that I'm heading. Many people want to emulate a home or office design from magazines or television. In their mind, they're convinced the same design concept can work in their space when it can't. There's nothing inherently wrong with wanting to emulate other beautiful spaces. However, not all interior spaces are equal. Most of us have seen houses that combine different designs that just don't work. The same applies when we think another's leadership style works for us. We'll talk more about this in a future chapter.

For now, perceptions like these are what psychiatrists and psychologists refer to as thinking traps or cognitive distortions. Along with several others, psychiatrists David D. Burns and Aaron T. Beck developed a list of what are described as thinking traps. Beck discovered that frequent negative automatic thoughts reveal a person's core beliefs. He explains that core beliefs are formed over lifelong experiences; we "feel" these beliefs to be true. Beck termed these cognitions "automatic thoughts."[1]

Cognition simply implies our perception of reality—how we interpret the world around us and ourselves, what we communicate to ourselves, our beliefs, our values, our behaviors, etc., as we saw earlier with Marie, Ben, Jerry, and Travis. In this chapter, we'll highlight some common thinking traps and show you how they can act as liabilities to leaders. Then we'll introduce a strategic intervention for undoing the associated behavior.

THINKING TRAP #1: TUNNEL VISION

Leaders fall into the tunnel vision trap when they're hell-bent on checking tasks off their to-do lists. They're recklessly determined to complete a task at any cost. The destination is fixed, and everything else is sacrificed for its achievement. Remember Travis? Sounds like him, doesn't it? Because of Travis' determined drive, he fell into the achievement trap as he focused on

CHAPTER 4: Recognizing The Traps & The Liabilities

his work over all else. While neck-deep in working, he sacrificed his emotional and strategic insight, causing him to fail to see the bigger picture.

Liabilities

- Losing sight of your vision for the company and floundering at execution
- Confusing your team about where everyone's headed
- Creating silos within the organization
- Offensive and curt behavior

THINKING TRAP #2: SOLO JUDGING

Leaders fall into the solo judging trap when they think no one can do the job as well as they can, so they separate from everyone in an attempt to do it all alone. They put unnecessary pressure on themselves, refusing to delegate for fear that their standards won't be met. Remember Marie from Chapter 3? She fell into this thinking trap. In her mind, her approach to work was far superior to her teammates. She eventually trapped herself in isolation, thinking she was the only one who cared about an effective work ethic and excellent performance.

Liabilities

- A disconnect and lack of trust between the leader and the team
- Marginalizing and not recognizing others for their efforts
- Putting an overwhelming amount of anxiety and stress on the leader

THINKING TRAP #3: IMAGE CONTROL

At times when a leader's reputation and influence are on the line, they can easily fall into the trap of concealing their mistakes or redirecting the blame. They are used to being in control, supported, and effective in every endeavor. They're similar to Jerry from Chapter 3. When things didn't go as he planned, in protecting his image, he found it safer to blame his colleagues instead of owning up to his shortcomings. Typically, this type of leadership produces disjointed teams with no clear strategic vision for growth. It's difficult for them to come together to solve critical issues, so problems ultimately get swept under the rug.

Liabilities

- Losing trust and confidence in the team
- Focusing on self rather than on solutions
- Compromising the company culture and morale

THINKING TRAP #4: RUSHED DECISIONS

Leaders can fall into the trap of making decisions that conflict with their own morals, values, and vision. They bypass their inner warning signs and unconsciously take action that doesn't quite click with what they originally wanted to accomplish. Sounds like Ben from the previous chapter, doesn't it? Over time, leaders who make decisions without thinking about the consequences often find themselves trapped between two fires, compromising their values in favor of moving ahead professionally. Then they have to spend a lot of time repairing the damage they have created in both their professional and personal relationships.

Liabilities

- Causing tension, frustration, and distrust within the organization
- Compromising loyalty and retention
- Questioning the leader's integrity

THINKING TRAP #5: FEELING COMFORTABLE

This is a dangerous trap (well, they all are). Leaders who relax when things are going well can fall into a routine that will trap them in thinking, "Now I can relax and pull back for a while." This type of thinking can easily and insidiously give you comfort—a cheap source of happiness—and cause you to overlook

CHAPTER 4: Recognizing The Traps & The Liabilities

growth opportunities as things appear to be going well. In the next chapter, Jackie is a clear example of this behavior. Leaders who are comfortable and complacent will eventually lose their drive to challenge the status quo. They're satisfied with not investing in their professional development. They stick to what they know and quickly dismiss ideas that do not appear to be a strategic fit, possibly leading to risk-averse behaviors.

Liabilities

- Falling behind on cultural and technological advancements
- Wavering growth of the organization
- Competing externally becomes a greater threat

THINKING TRAP #6: STRATEGIC MYOPIA

When leaders fail to see past what's currently on their radar, they can fall into the kind of trap that prevents them from seeing the forest when they're surrounded by trees. They only see things clearly in the short term. This strategic myopia or short-sightedness impedes their effective long-term planning and execution. They're stuck in the present. They focus on the short term to the detriment of the long term. This could be a problem because investors may see the company as a potential risk.

Liabilities

- Obstructing your preparation for future opportunities and challenges
- Separating and turning away the culture
- Immobilizing the appropriate resources where they are needed

THINKING TRAP #7: CATASTROPHIZING

Leaders with this distortion typically believe that something will be far worse than it is. Even though they're determined to succeed, they can fall into the trap of continually playing it safe, which leads to risk-averse behaviors.

LEAD2FLOURISH

While feeling afraid to make a mistake, this kind of trap can hinder leaders from accepting new ideas, thus causing them to shy away from taking up challenging initiatives. They often regret past failures and view them as letdowns, serious personal flaws, or catastrophes.

Liabilities

- Limiting your growth potential and the team's
- Inhibiting you from preparing for future opportunities and challenges
- Inhibiting team members from taking action

As you can see, we are essentially unconscious of our own choices and behaviors even though we think we're fully aware of them. Behavior myths and misinformation like these are what keep us from leading from our highest selves.

Your Childhood May Have Some Clues

Becoming reacquainted with our childhood beliefs is a way to understand how we think as an adult. The most prominent views on this come from cognitive neuroscientist Dr. Caroline Leaf. From her book, *Switch on Your Brain*: "We are wired to consciously choose to bring the memory into consciousness where it becomes plastic enough to be changed. In practicing this daily, we are wiring the healthy new thoughts deeply into the mind." This is how we reverse self-limiting thoughts and behaviors.[2] And this is how we fulfill the highest act of leadership—self-awareness.

My Theory Confirmed

Years ago, I was a guest on a podcast, sharing ways to design your best life that impressed a lady listening in Australia. She later hired me to be her coach. Carrying a lot of anger, presumptions, and animosity toward her colleagues

CHAPTER 4: Recognizing The Traps & The Liabilities

and family hurt her career. Needing to protect her ego played into her behaviors and decisions, both personally and professionally. But she wanted to fearlessly do a higher quality of work that was more focused on both her and the company's goals. Still, her *fighting-ego* had her locked into a counter-productive pattern which was limiting her potential. Working with her confirmed my theory that childhood experiences do affect our beliefs as an adult and ultimately impact our performance, wellbeing, and ability to flourish.

In using cognitive behavior and emotional regulation research, a useful corollary for getting to the source of negative behaviors is recalling the experience or event that caused us to think a particular way or believe a particular thing. Psychologist Albert Ellis developed *Rational Emotive Behavior Therapy* (REBT) to help people better deal with the irrational thinking and beliefs associated with adverse experiences. REBT increases our self-awareness by teaching us to identify, challenge, and replace self-defeating beliefs with healthier ones that promote emotional wellbeing and goal achievement.

SIX PRINCIPLES OF RECOGNIZING AND UNDOING EGO-DRIVEN BEHAVIOR PATTERNS

Keep the following principles in mind as you begin recognizing ego-driven behavior patterns. The aim is to process your past to not relive your pains, but to find intrinsic motivation in the face of adversity and reconnect with your sincerity to make a larger difference. These steps follow in a simple ABCDEF order: *Address, Belief, Consequence, Dispute, Exchange, Forgive.*

1. **Address:** Address the activating childhood event(s) or experience(s) as an entity in itself.

What happened? Let's look again at Marie from Chapter 3. In her situation, she experienced the shame and fear associated with her father's alcoholism that, in her mind, shamed the family. In her prideful way of thinking, Marie needed to erase that scar and substitute it with excellence and professionalism.

Here's what you need to do:

Find a quiet place to recall and review as much as possible the details from your childhood experiences. Explore your reactions to these experiences. Make a note of every emotion associated with every experience. This doesn't have to be painful. Remember that, in the end, it will come to a beneficial conclusion.

2. **Belief:** Belief is the conviction you've carried resulting from your childhood experience.

   Marie believed love was something to be earned because she wasn't valued as a child. Have you developed any beliefs because of what you've experienced as a child? What happened?

Here's what you need to do:

Ask yourself: "What is my negative self-talk?" "Am I trapped in an irrational way of thinking?" "What negative beliefs am I clinging to?" "How am I interpreting these beliefs?" Write these down. Notice particularly which belief prompts the strongest emotion and reaction (the behavior).

3. **Consequence:** What was the consequence of your beliefs, e.g., thoughts, feelings, emotions, behavior?

   In Marie's situation, she felt dishonorable, ashamed, and unloved. Give yourself some options and explore your feelings.

Here's what you need to do:

Name specifically the emotions that you strongly feel and write them down. (For example, sad, angry, insulted, hopeless, heartbroken, betrayed, hateful, and the like). Do the sensations or emotions you're experiencing right now connect with one or more experiences in your past? Does it give you an insight into the root of a negative, limiting belief about yourself? Ask yourself, "In what ways did this feeling hold me back?" You need complete awareness of each feeling that is controlling your mind right now. This will give you a deeper self-awareness, your tool for the outcome that you seek.

CHAPTER 4: Recognizing The Traps & The Liabilities

4. **Dispute**: Now that you've completed your inner research, it's time to dispute the experience or event and support it with the facts.

    Marie was right that her father's alcoholism disgraced the family, but she disputed that it was a reason to judge others. The facts were clear; her team members were smart and capable. Stick with this step. Although it may seem hard, it's doable.

Here's what you need to do:

First, it's essential that you face your ego and tell it that the beliefs and thinking traps you've carried because of your childhood experiences are simply not truths. Ask yourself, "What are my counter-thoughts?" "What realistic and grounding statement can I use instead?" "What is a reality-based alternative way of thinking?"

5. **Exchange**: You are now ready to exchange the limiting belief and behavior for optimistic and inspiring ones.

    Yes, you can do this. Science shows that you are wired for love and optimism. Marie exchanged her negative, solo-judging thinking for an understanding that her father's alcoholism problem wasn't hers to fix. She realized that the experience was misinterpreted. You're capable of standing outside yourself, observing your thinking, consulting with your consciousness, changing the limiting thought, and growing healthy, positive thoughts. When you do this, your brain responds with a positive neurochemical rush and structural change that will improve your intellect, health, and peace. You will experience soul harmony.[3]

Here's what you need to do:

In her book, *Who Switched Off My Brain?*, Dr. Carol Leaf talks about intentionally meditating on honorable, right, wholesome, lovely, and admirable experiences, which allows your positive neurons to fire up those neurons for positive thinking. Recognize that good experiences are sinking into you.

Dr. Leaf recommends we do this: Meditate on positive experiences for ten minutes a day for at least twenty-one days. As Dr. Leaf's book shows, intentional meditation on positive experiences helps you wire healthy new thoughts more deeply into the mind. Your mind shapes your world. You're no longer rehearsing negative events or limiting beliefs.

The neurons now aren't getting enough negative signals and are firing apart, which destroys the emotion (*fighting-ego*) that was attached to the childhood event.[4]

6. **Forgive:** This last principle is a tool that keeps groups, teams, and families together.

I included forgiveness with Ellis' REBT model because it seals the deal. I instructed my Australian client to make the conscious decision to forgive for something she'd experienced as a child. After doing this, she told me, "I feel like I have more freedom and control. It's easy for me to be empathic and compassionate toward my teammates at work, and I'm happier than I've ever been in my life!"

Likewise, Marie first forgave her deceased father and then forgave herself for her behavior. Here's a piece of advice directly from Marie: "Acknowledge your fears. You cannot change what you do not acknowledge." Building on her own life experiences with forgiveness, Dr. Shawne Duperon says, "Forgiveness is a bold leadership skill."[5] Unconscious suffering brings the opportunity to release and forgive. And Yale psychologist Molly Crockett said, "The brain forms social impressions in a way that can enable forgiveness."[6]

Here's what you need to do:

Let go of the need for revenge and release negative thoughts. Remember, forgiveness is something you do for yourself, not others.[7] Now that you've unearthed the childhood experience causing the limiting beliefs and behaviors, it's time to forgive the experience and everyone within the experience, including yourself. Who's right or wrong is irrelevant.

CHAPTER 4: Recognizing The Traps & The Liabilities

Make a conscious decision to forgive whomever you feel is responsible. If someone else is responsible for your hurt, try seeing things from their perspective. Take ownership of your decision to let go of the hurt and move forward. Steve Maraboli, the author of *Unapologetically You*, reveals, "The truth is, unless you let go, unless you forgive yourself, unless you forgive the situation, unless you realize that the situation is over, you cannot move forward."

Lead2Flourish Keys

1. A leader who manages large teams and must make crucial decisions for the organization has to maintain a sturdy mental balance to retain leadership success.
2. Undoing what has held you back can improve your judgment and help you identify opportunities for professional development and personal growth.
3. Your brain may have stamps from the past, but it's being rewired by your positive expectation of the future.
4. The seven thinking traps most common to leaders reveal that you're essentially blind to your own choices and behaviors even though you think that you're fully aware of them.

Questions for Reflection

1. What can you do now to bring awareness to unhelpful belief patterns?
2. Which of the seven thinking traps reflects your behavior?
3. Who can you ask for honest feedback about how you're perceived by others?
4. What are your intrinsic motivators for recognizing and taming unhelpful belief patterns?
5. What's your plan to diminish the liabilities?

Designing a Lead2Flourish Plan – Recognizing the Traps and Liabilities

Reflecting on what you've learned in this chapter, <u>design a plan to change the impact of unhelpful belief patterns that hijack your behavior, wellbeing, and ability to flourish.</u>

1. The unhelpful thoughts and belief patterns I'm facing are:
2. I've decided to commit to:
3. The reasons I've made this decision are:
4. Potential *fighting-ego* hurdles:
5. One small change I can make now is:
6. I will introduce "undoing unhelpful belief patterns" to my organization beginning with…
7. My timeline:

Next, I will open a Pandora's Box and expose the behavior myths and misinformation that keep you from leading from your highest self.

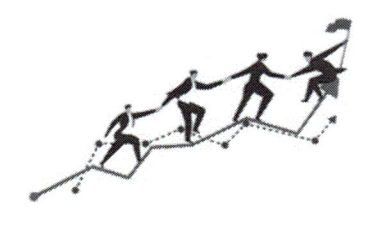

CHAPTER 5

MYTHS & MISINFORMATION: RECOGNIZING THE DAMAGES

Pandora's Box of Myths

Over the course of my two-plus decades in corporate leadership, I've had many opportunities to see effective and ineffective behaviors that impacted leadership results. Certainly, I've fallen prey to some of the myths that I talk about in this chapter and suffered the consequences. So, I write this chapter not only from a scientific perspective but with the advantage of hindsight.

Much is taught about "what to do" and little about "what not to do" as a leader. Unfortunately, doing a lot of the things that leaders are taught can trigger the thoughts that open the Pandora's Box of myths and misinformation like these:

1. Overthinking (ruminating) is problem-solving
2. Multitasking is productivity
3. Feedback is criticism
4. Work and life must be balanced

Einstein said insanity is doing the same thing over and over, expecting different results. Together, we will break the insanity cycle by exposing and gaining more clarity about the behavior myths we've been led to accept.

BEHAVIOR MYTH #1: OVERTHINKING IS PROBLEM-SOLVING

Getting Out of Your Head

Getting out of your way is crucial to flourishing. But you also need to get out of your head. We're all thinkers. We talk to ourselves. Our fast-paced, overly self-analytical culture is pushing us to spend countless hours thinking about negative ideas, feelings, and experiences. Psychologist Dr. Susan Nolen-Hoeksema calls this overthinking. Our thinking patterns and words determine the direction and quality of our lives. This part of the chapter examines how the ego pushes us to unconsciously overthink, upsetting our wellbeing and affecting work performance.

Many believe that overthinking is problem-solving or self-reflecting. However, problem-solving and self-reflection are purposeful. Problem-solving involves approaching a problem with a solid process while thinking about a creative solution. Self-reflection involves learning something about ourselves or gaining a new perspective on a situation. Time spent developing creative solutions or learning about our behavior is productive.

Conversely, overthinking is counterproductive. When we overthink, we are dwelling on the problem—causing us to feel bad as we think about all the things we have no control over. We can't gain good insight this way.

CHAPTER 5: Myths & Misinformation: Recognizing The Damages

This was discovered in a UK study: When certain parts of our brain and cognitive processes are quiet, we're more creative. According to this study, overthinking can lead to a "mental rut" and essentially cause us to get stuck.1 Think about how a computer browser slows down or gets stuck from the stress of having an increasing number of opened tabs. The browser takes longer to display the pages.

Much the same way, the stress of overthinking can slow the process of regeneration of our brain cells, draining us of mental energy. When we overthink and stress ourselves out, stress hormones, like cortisol and adrenaline get released into the body. Over time, that constant release of cortisol can be depleting and cause burnout.2 And just like the computer with too many opened tabs, the brain is limited—we can only pay attention to about seven bits of information at a time.

I wanted to hear from other executives and business owners. What was going on in their heads? How were they affected? Let's look at Paul's and Gina's stories.

Meet Paul

Paul is a forty-seven-year-old environmental engineer. He's been married to Doris for eleven years, and they have three sons. Paul takes pleasure in his work. He's honored to provide a service that helps people enhance their quality of life. Plus, there's great camaraderie among his teammates. Traveling to and monitoring different job sites keeps everything exciting and fresh. But Paul's demeanor suddenly changed after receiving a much-deserved promotion to a senior-level position. The new position requires him to be in the office most of the time involved with overseeing design and planning. If we were able to listen to Paul's thoughts while looking over his charts, we'd hear him replaying this conversation:

LEAD2FLOURISH

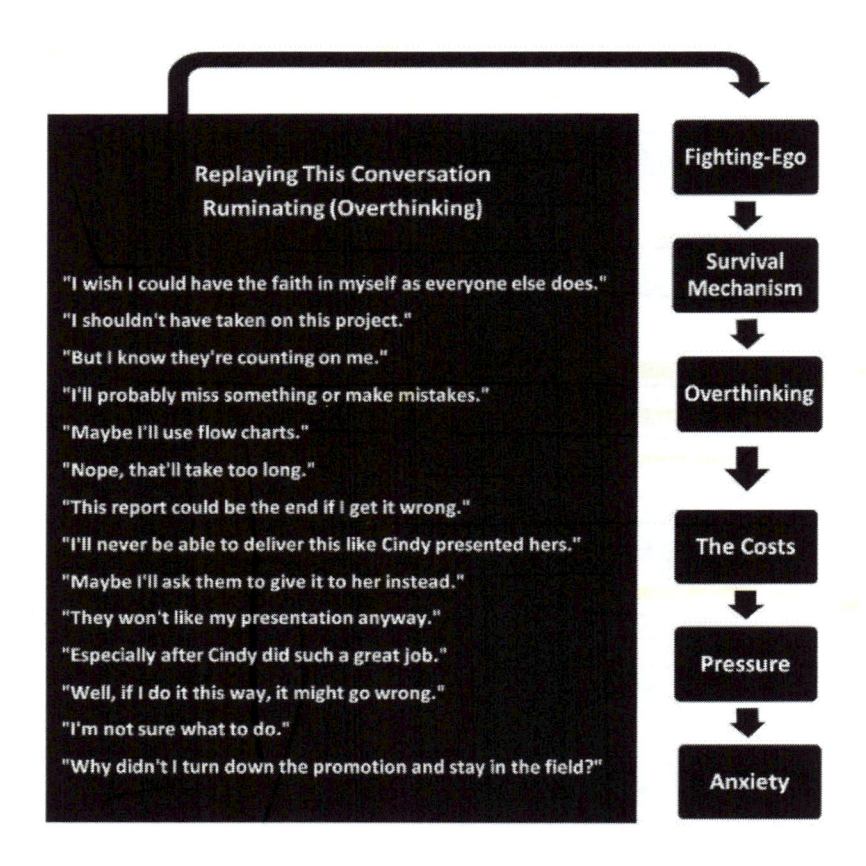

Replaying This Conversation Ruminating (Overthinking)

"I wish I could have the faith in myself as everyone else does."
"I shouldn't have taken on this project."
"But I know they're counting on me."
"I'll probably miss something or make mistakes."
"Maybe I'll use flow charts."
"Nope, that'll take too long."
"This report could be the end if I get it wrong."
"I'll never be able to deliver this like Cindy presented hers."
"Maybe I'll ask them to give it to her instead."
"They won't like my presentation anyway."
"Especially after Cindy did such a great job."
"Well, if I do it this way, it might go wrong."
"I'm not sure what to do."
"Why didn't I turn down the promotion and stay in the field?"

Fighting-Ego → Survival Mechanism → Overthinking → The Costs → Pressure → Anxiety → (loop back to Fighting-Ego)

Although Paul doesn't realize it, his main problem isn't getting the project finished. Neither is it competing with Cindy for praise and recognition. Paul's problem is being pulled by the strings of his *fighting-ego*. He doesn't have an accurate and balanced profile of who he is. He's replaying conversations over in his head, running different scenarios, wondering how to handle a non-existent situation. He criticizes himself for potential mistakes he hasn't even made that are causing him much distress. And worst of all, he becomes too paralyzed to take action. Paul's real problem is his survival mechanism—analysis paralysis. The more he thinks, the worse he feels. Now he's stuck in his feelings of misery and anxiety. His clouded judgment prevents him from taking positive action.

CHAPTER 5: Myths & Misinformation: Recognizing The Damages

Meet Gina

Gina had a similar problem. Gina is a thirty-nine-year-old controller and accounting manager at a luxe department store. She recently got engaged to Rick, whom she dated for three years. Gina lives with her two active puppies: Sammy, the Golden Retriever, and Peaches, the Irish Setter. The three of them run together every morning and evening. Her work and social life couldn't be better. This is Gina's second management position at a high-end store, and she's happy there. She works closely with the financial management team, and her dedication and engagement are frequently recognized and rewarded.

After working every evening on an arduous assignment for the past six weeks, Gina finalized the project on Friday evening before Christmas. All she could think about was having a relaxing weekend at home with her puppies. As she's shutting down her computer for the day, the financial executive calls to say:

> "Gina, it appears that you've overlooked an error in one of your reports."
>
> "An error?" she reacts. "Gee, what exactly did I miss?"
>
> "How could I have been so careless?" "I'm so sorry this happened," were her thoughts while continuing to explain what possibly could have occurred.
>
> "We can go over this on Monday," he said. "Have a good weekend."

Gina couldn't let it go. Her self-talk was saying, *"Have a good weekend? How do I have a good weekend after screwing up my biggest assignment of the year?"* She allowed the error to gnaw at her, rehashing it over and over in her mind and dwelling on how life can be so unfair. Repeatedly thinking about where the error could be and how embarrassed she was, her ego prevented her from having a relaxed weekend. Instead, she had a lousy, sleepless one. And her fiancé and puppies suffered through it with her.

Paul and Gina are *overthinkers*. The problem lies in their unawareness of this. Overthinking comes in two different forms, with the same stressful effects. Paul is negatively ruminating about what could happen in the future, and Gina's negativity bias is brooding on what happened in the past. And they both outwardly demonstrate it with negative self-talk.

Many of us believe that when we feel down, we should try to focus inwardly. We tend to evaluate our feelings and our situation, looking for self-insight and solutions that might ultimately resolve our problems. Numerous studies over the past two decades have shown that, on the contrary, overthinking ushers in a host of adverse consequences: It sustains or worsens sadness, fosters negatively biased thinking, impairs a person's ability to solve problems, saps motivation, and interferes with concentration and initiative. Moreover, although people have a strong sense that they are gaining insight into themselves and their problems during their ruminations, this is rarely the case. What they do gain is a distorted, pessimistic perspective on their lives.[3]

Overthinking (Ruminating) Concerns

Dr. Susan Nolen-Hoeksema's ground-breaking research discovered that when you ruminate while in a depressed mood, you remember more negative things that happened to you in the past, you interpret situations in your current life more negatively, and you're more hopeless about the future.

Ruminating for an extended time can drive away your social support and put you on the fast track to feeling helpless. Specifically, it paralyzes your problem-solving skills.[4] The research of Dr. Laura Price found that your gut feeling or instinct gets overridden because you have so much other input, and you may end up not making the choices that are right for you at that moment.[5]

CHAPTER 5: Myths & Misinformation: Recognizing The Damages

Negativity Bias Concerns

Scientists tell us that we have a *negativity bias,* which refers to the asymmetrical way we perceive the negative and the positive. Studies have found that the brain generally reacts more to a negative stimulus than to an equally intense positive one. You've probably noticed that focusing your thoughts and feelings on negative aspects of an issue cloud your thinking. This makes it more difficult to accurately assess circumstances when making critical decisions and reduces our ability to handle issues with emotional intelligence.[6] So, what's the cause?

According to psychologist and *New York Times* bestselling author Rick Hanson, the effects of the negativity bias are "a growing sensitivity to stress, upset, and other negative experiences; a tendency toward pessimism, regret and resentment; and long shadows cast by old pain."[7]

Ruminating and negativity bias can be particularly harmful to leaders. Why? First thing, a leader's mood can be contagious. Negative emotions, such as frustration, anxiety, and fear, can transmit easily from a leader to their team. Another view is a leader's negative emotions can loom large and discourage people, narrow their thinking, and act as a dimmer switch for performance.

The good news is that we aren't prisoners of overthinking. We can raise our awareness when our thinking roams and slips into pessimism or lack of enthusiasm. We can take steps to manage our frame of mind so we can harness the power of positivity for growth and success. Remember, leaders can't lead others if they don't first lead themselves.

How?

Change your outlook on a negative situation or experience by looking on the bright side. My grandmother would say this a lot. I know you've heard this before and may even believe it's just a cliché, but it's an evidence-based approach to countering known problematic thought patterns. Parallel to looking on the bright side, renowned psychologist and Wharton professor Adam Grant encourage us to rethink (not overthink) situations and wishes more leaders from all industries would think like scientists.[8] In his newest book, *Think Again,* he explains how scientists:

- Are constantly aware of the limits of their understanding
- Doubt what they know
- Are curious about what they don't know
- Update their views based on new data

You cannot control the events and circumstances of life, but you can control your reactions to those events. Controlling your reactions increases your chances of changing your brain. Before you can put an end to overthinking, you must recognize when and why you're doing it.

FIVE PRINCIPLES OF EXCAVATING THE OVERTHINKING MINDSET

Also referred to as cognitive reframing, you can shift your mindset so that you're able to look at a situation, person, or relationship from a different perspective. Did you know studies confirm that looking on the bright side or reframing an otherwise grim situation builds optimism and resilience? My grandmother knew to do this, and she wasn't a scientist. When you catch yourself overthinking, take time to explore the following process.

1. *Recognize why you're overthinking*

Do you remember how Paul thought about himself and his job? His *fighting-ego* convinced him he'd made the wrong decision to accept the promotion. Thinking his career would be in jeopardy if he couldn't outperform Cindy inhibited him from taking business initiatives. But the true reason for this unconscious behavior was lacking an accurate and balanced profile of who he was. Once he recognized why he ruminated, it was easier for him to access its accuracy.

CHAPTER 5: Myths & Misinformation: Recognizing The Damages

Here's what you need to do:

Like Paul, your *fighting-ego* may have convinced you to remain mediocre or stuck by triggering you to believe negative stories about yourself. Pay attention to what's going on in your life as you engage in this behavior. Is it when you need to make a tough life decision? Is It when you're faced with your insecurities or fears? Or is it when you become emotionally drained or stressed? Nail it down to the why.

2. *Assess the accuracy of your thinking*

I attended a conference and heard the speaker say, "Always doubt the doubt." Though this was many years ago, the impact of that instruction was so strong and powerful that I've never forgotten it. So, I adopted it as a measure to assess the accuracy of my thinking. I've learned to either believe or doubt the outcome of where my thinking is taking me.

Here's what you need to do:

Ask yourself where your thoughts and beliefs come from. Analyze it. You already know if your thoughts and beliefs are grounded in opinions or based on facts. At least I hope you do. But if it's just your opinion, then it most likely falls under the category of doubt. If it's based on a fact, you can assess that it's accurate. Now you can doubt the doubt that's contrary to this fact.

3. *Make amendments*

Did you know you can modify your thoughts to those that make you feel like your life is enjoyable, worthwhile, and/or meaningful? It would've been very easy for Gina to undo her thinking about what went wrong that day by coming up with at least five situations of when she got it right. Can you recognize how the energy in letting go helps you to converge into a constructive state of mind?

LEAD2FLOURISH

Here's what you need to do:

When you start telling yourself these unhelpful stories, replace them with encouraging ones, like "This isn't as big as it appears, and I'm in full control of my emotions." All Gina needed to do was reframe her thoughts to bring them in line with her enjoyable, worthwhile, and/or meaningful weekend goals. Her executive already led the way for her. She could've reframed the thought to "It was good of the executive to catch the error before the reports left the building." I want you to understand the ease of amending your unhelpful thoughts by simply reframing them to align with your goals. This is how you look on the bright side of it.

4. See the bright side

Had Gina looked on the bright side of the situation, there was nothing to be concerned about. She would've felt how wonderful it is to engage in positive mind searching. What's your situation that you can see from the bright side? Consider what you gained from it.

Here's what you need to do:

Ask yourself questions that allow you to amend your overthinking behavior and move forward. Come up with at least three positive things that can come out of a recent difficulty. For example, some positives to coming out of missing an important deadline may include permitting yourself to be human because everyone makes mistakes, or finding the ability to control and overcome the anxiety and discomfort of being overwhelmed.

5. Savor the bright side

While both Paul and Gina had a human moment or two, it didn't mean that there was no space for brighter things to happen. By intentionally giving their attention to positive, more useful facts, reframing their thoughts, and prolonging the supporting feelings, they can buffer against floundering outcomes and enable

CHAPTER 5: Myths & Misinformation: Recognizing The Damages

flourishing. You can activate the behavior of savoring by attending, appreciating, and enhancing positive experiences that occur in your life.

Here's what you need to do:

Give yourself ample time—at least 20-30 seconds—to fully enjoy the reframed thought. What you're doing is consciously experiencing a pleasant way of thinking. Can you feel the freedom in recognizing that being human means sometimes making mistakes? By elongating your positive sensations of savoring the bright side, you allow more neurons to fire and wire together in response to this positive stimulus. This solidifies the experience in your memory. I want you to remember that you're in full control of your reality.

Practicing these five principles every day will highlight positive aspects of life and the upside of challenging situations, moving you away from overthinking and fixating on the downsides. And besides, if it feels right, why overthink it?

Lead2Flourish Keys

1. Overthinking sustains or worsens sadness, fosters negatively biased thinking, and impairs a person's ability to solve problems.
2. Overthinking or ruminating causes you to expend considerable emotional energy that drains the resources to live a flourishing life.
3. Focusing your thoughts and feelings on unhelpful or discouraging aspects of an issue makes it more difficult to accurately assess circumstances when making critical decisions and reduces your ability to handle issues with emotional intelligence.
4. Negative emotions can transmit easily from a leader to their team, discourage people, narrow their thinking, and act as a dimmer switch on performance.

LEAD2FLOURISH

5. When you slip into negative thinking, you can take steps to manage your frame of mind and harness the power of positivity for growth and success.
6. Before you can put an end to overthinking, you must recognize when and why you're doing it.
7. By assessing the accuracy of your thinking, adapting to meaningful thoughts, and savoring the bright side and positive aspects of life, you allow more neurons to fire and wire together in response to this positive stimulus.
8. Looking on the bright side or reframing an otherwise grim situation builds optimism and resilience.

Questions for Reflection

1. Does overthinking give me a false sense of control?
2. What vulnerable feelings am I hiding in my tendency to overthink?
3. How can I move from overthinking to a courageous, strategic, risk-taking thinking style?

Designing a Lead2Flourish Plan – The Costs of Overthinking

Reflecting on what you've learned in this segment, practice recognizing your overthinking tendencies and design a plan for overcoming your overthinking tendencies.

1. I tend to overthink when:
2. I've decided to set practical overthinking boundaries by:
3. The reasons I've made these decisions are:
4. Potential fighting-ego hurdles:
5. How can I intentionally seek solutions and constructively engage in self-Reflection?

CHAPTER 5: Myths & Misinformation: Recognizing The Damages

6. How will I introduce "overthinking is not problem-solving" to my organization?
7. My timeline:

BEHAVIOR MYTH #2:
MULTITASKING IS TIME MANAGEMENT

Ego-Driven Performance

If you find yourself searching through emails while talking on the phone, participating in conference calls while driving, reading while listening to music, or texting while in meetings, then you're multitasking. Multitasking is trying to do two or more cognitive things at the same time. But Stanford researchers say even trying may impair your cognitive control. We often believe this behavior helps us to keep a finger on the pulse of our productivity and the company's growth. But it's the ego that's driving this behavior. Despite our best intentions, we get pulled into doing multiple tasks at the expense of efficiency.

As we do more, we hope to rise in the ranks and acquire more power. We then feel that we have to do even more with the time we have. People see us as the high performer who always gets things done. This pleases the ego, and like any addiction, we like how the spotlight and attention make us feel. We want more and more. But multitasking is a myth and more like a productivity illusion. We're doing what researchers call "task-switching." This is a skill that leaders should never develop.

Getting to the Brain of Task-switching Behavior

Earl K. Miller, the Picower Professor of Neuroscience at the Massachusetts Institute of Technology, explains that our brain has a very limited bandwidth to process new information. It can handle a very small number of thoughts at one time. Contrary to what people think, it isn't possible to think about two things at once. The best we can manage is switching back and forth between two things quickly. The brain is forced to switch between multiple cognitive tasks as these tasks use the same part of the brain. There are several things you should know about task-switching behavior:

- **Every time we switch our focus from one thing to another, there's a switch cost.** That start-stop-start process is hard on us. Our brain stumbles a bit, and it requires time to get back to where it was before it was distracted. Rather than saving time, it costs time, even microseconds. It's less efficient, we make more mistakes, and over time, it can sap our energy.

- **We cannot think as deeply about something when we're being distracted every few minutes.** And thinking deeply is where real insights come from. The human brain evolved in an environment where there was much less information, and any potential information could be helpful as a means of survival. Today we're in a very different environment. Our brains weren't designed for overloads of information. We're wired to find information rewarding, yet our brains want to seek out all this information even though it is maladaptive.[9]

- **We sacrifice the quality of our attention.** According to Simons & Chabris, we perceive and remember only those objects and details that receive focused attention. The poor focus of attention and lack of quality in our thoughts are the complete opposite of how the brain is designed to function and cause a level of brain damage. Task-switching also creates patterns of flightiness and lack of concentration that, unfortunately, are often erroneously labeled ADD and ADHD. This opens us up to shallow and weak judgments and decisions, and it results in passive mindlessness.[10]

CHAPTER 5: Myths & Misinformation: Recognizing The Damages

- **Task-switching** involves several parts of our brain. Brain scans during task-switching show activity in four major areas: the *prefrontal cortex* is involved in shifting and focusing our attention and selecting which task to do when. The *posterior parietal* lobe activates rules for each task we switch to. The *anterior cingulate gyrus* monitors errors. And the *premotor cortex* is preparing for us to move in some way. We now know that the multiple tasks that we're attending to are sharing brain time. Interestingly, this coincides with a Stanford University study that shows how those who task-switch are indeed worse performers and struggle because they can't filter out irrelevant information, resulting in slowing down the completion of the cognitive task at hand. The study also reveals that task-switching adds stress to our daily lives and negatively affects our mood, motivation, and productivity.[11]

Executives must wear many hats each day, toggling between different apps for team projects and other apps for organizing work-related tasks. You're responding to updates in your team's collaboration platform while writing a report. Having to navigate from one app to another, you lose your train of thought in the process. Then you seek out ways to manage stress to boost performance and mood, while task-switching may be the problem.

SIX PRINCIPLES OF UNDOING TASK-SWITCHING BEHAVIOR

There's a current trend in neuroscience toward mindfulness-based practices and training. Although a lot of studies talk about Eastern mediation techniques, what they come down to every time is the ancient biblical principle of focus reflection. It's deep, intellectual, disciplined thinking with attention regulation, body awareness, emotional regulation, and a sense of self that positively changes us. The following series of steps will help you to cope with all the input and distractions you have in your life, especially at work:

1. **Recognize it**

    The first step to changing any behavior is awareness. Self-awareness is a skill that, like a muscle, needs a good workout to stay strong and flexible.

    Here's what you need to do:

    Accept the fundamental fact that the mind can only do one thing at a time. Keep in mind that this can be challenging because your brain is addicted to the dopamine rush generated by task-switching. For this reason, you must be cleverer than the temptation. For example, each time you feel the urge to switch tasks, attack the ego-driven behavior. Say out loud: "I'm not doing this anymore. My focus is on one task at a time!" Your words create your world.

2. **Prioritize prioritizing**

    Get excited about this step and make it an energy-intensive activity.

    Here's what you need to do:

    Schedule the most attention-rich tasks when you have a fresh and alert mind. For example, honor the 80/20 rule. 20% of the work you do gives 80% of the impact and effectiveness. Focus on identifying the 20% of your tasks that are effective. Plan to tackle only those that you can manage for the day and do them one at a time.

3. **Simplify and divide**

    When you figure out how to take the complex or complicated and simplify it so you can get it done, you'll have time and energy to move on to the next task.

    Here's what you need to do:

    Approximate and focus on an idea's most important elements. For example, group information into chunks whenever there is too much to take in. Practice doing the most energy-consuming and difficult tasks before the easier ones.

CHAPTER 5: Myths & Misinformation: Recognizing The Damages

4. *Catch yourself*

Very few tasks that you do are entirely conscious. Your *fighting-ego* will want to pull and push you to unconsciously shift from one task to another. Catch yourself by shifting the task into your conscious mind to deal with it.

Here's what you need to do:

When you find yourself doing two things at once, immediately stop. Put tasks into a neat and functional order. For example, before going to bed, identify and journal one or two important things that you want to accomplish the following day. Those are the tasks you'll handle first. This reduces the anxious drive to do more and will make it easier to resist task-switching.

5. *Center on focus time*

Give yourself specific focus time to work on one task. This technique has worked well for my clients and me.

Here's what you need to do:

Let's say, for example, that you have a report to review among your other day-to-day responsibilities. Block off from one hour to perhaps a half-day and only work on the report. Before you start, close your door, or find a quiet place to be alone. Turn off the audio and visual cues built into the devices that alert you to the presence of more information. You'll notice how energized this makes you feel.

6. *Leverage private time*

The executive region of the brain that's involved in controlling behavior, intellectual ability, and memory is called the *prefrontal cortex*. Creativity research tells us that this region is central to creativity. You'll never solve problems if your *prefrontal cortex* doesn't get quiet time to work on assimilating information.

LEAD2FLOURISH

Here's what you need to do:

Set aside time in your day to do nothing that will tax your brain. Go for a walk, exercise, meditate, listen to music, visit a museum, or gaze in nature. You'll find that setting aside quiet time like this energizes you to get more work done.

Remember that mental clutter keeps you tethered to task-switching. To think clearly, you must become a **FAT thinker**—thinking *Flexibly, Accurately,* and *Thoroughly*. Evaluating your thinking in a FAT approach will improve your emotional state and your behavior.[12]

Lead2Flourish Keys

1. Every time you switch your focus from one thing to another, there's a switch cost.
2. While multitasking or task-switching impairs your cognitive control, it also inhibits your productivity and the company's growth.
3. It's far more efficient to fully focus for 90 to 120 minutes, take a true break, and then fully focus on the next activity.
4. Task-switching can give executives an egocentric illusion of being seen as the high performer who always gets things done to rise in the ranks and acquire more power.
5. Contrary to what people think, it isn't possible to think about two things at once.

Questions for Reflection

1. Think about the times you switched tasks within a day or worked on more than one task simultaneously. How productive were you?
2. When on a conference or casual call, how often did you check your

CHAPTER 5: Myths & Misinformation: Recognizing The Damages

email or social media? How often did you ask the speaker to repeat what was said? How often did you fog out of the conversation?
3. How do you react when you have several tasks to complete in a day?
4. Task-switching confuses our ability to do either task effectively. Reflect on how the following may have affected you:

- Total productivity can be reduced by up to 40 percent.
- An IQ can drop by around 10 points.
- It's difficult to retain new information while multitasking.
- More errors are made than if the same tasks are done with all our focus.

5. Can I downright multitask efficiently?

Designing a Lead2Flourish Plan – Undoing the Multitasking Behavior

Reflecting on what you've learned in this segment, practice recognizing multitasking as a mental overload that can result in a catastrophe. Design a plan that increases your focus and performance.

1. The task-switching behaviors I'm facing are:
2. I've decided to commit to:
3. The reasons I've made this decision are:
4. Potential *fighting-ego* hurdles:
5. I will boost my efficiency by avoiding multitasking by:
6. I introduce the fact that "multitasking is a myth" to my organization by:
7. My timeline:

BEHAVIOR MYTH #3:
FEEDBACK IS CRITICISM

Be Like Liz

Now that we've unpacked the multitasking myth, let's turn our attention to challenging another myth that executives often fall for: the idea that feedback is criticism. Jackie had many achievements to boast about; however, her take on feedback would cause her to slow down.

Jackie's department grew rapidly as well as her work responsibilities. She often worked late to meet demanding deadlines. To make things run more smoothly, she felt that an open-door policy would make it easier for everyone. The purpose was to create honest dialogue and respect where colleagues were free to talk with her and offer their feedback. They told her that though her work quality was stellar, her public presentations were boring.

A couple of months later, Jackie noticed that people were having discussions among themselves instead of coming directly to her. She talked about this with Liz, an executive from another department. During their conversation, Jackie discovered that there was a problem with how she reacted to their honest feedback. Jackie saw their honest feedback as criticism, so they stopped coming to her. Jackie believed that her effectiveness should be measured by her results and should speak volumes. Liz encouraged Jackie to loosen up and not take it personally.

I invite you to be like Liz. She understands how receiving and acting on feedback is a vital ingredient in the development of leaders in today's business world. No matter how well leaders are performing at work, regardless of their level, we *unconsciously* tend to dread feedback and fear performance reviews. While many are trained in the art of giving feedback to teams, the question is, how do we avoid reacting shamefully and respond effectively when we're on the receiving end?

CHAPTER 5: Myths & Misinformation: Recognizing The Damages

The Breakfast of Champions

Feedback is a powerful tool for giving us insight into our blind spots, a deeper understanding of performance improvement, and direction on developing talent or guiding promotions, as well as boosting the bottom line. According to researcher and consultant Ken Blanchard, "Feedback is the breakfast of champions."

If you want to flourish in leadership and be successful, you need quality feedback. The engagement and performance of our teams can hinge on how we receive and interpret feedback. People's helpful opinions can also have a profound effect on our growth and development. Upon receiving the feedback, do what Jackie did and talk it over with someone trustworthy and not in a role to evaluate your performance.

The best leaders ask for feedback, according to leadership consultants Jack Zenger and Joseph Folkman. In their recent study of 51,896 executives, for example, those who ranked at the bottom 10% in asking for feedback (that's to say, they asked for feedback less often than 90% of their peers) were rated at the 15th percentile in overall leadership effectiveness. On the other hand, leaders who ranked in the top 10% in asking for feedback were rated, on average, at the 86th percentile in overall leadership effectiveness. As we can see, research clearly shows the advantage of receiving feedback on an ongoing basis.[13]

So Why the Feedback Phobia?

Let's return to Jackie's story, who viewed her colleagues' feedback as criticism.

After initiating her open-door policy and hearing her colleagues' opinions, people began noticing how Jackie's demeanor had shifted. The once go-getter and deadline-buster Jackie had suddenly slowed down. While she'd talked to Liz about how badly the feedback stung, she became keenly unhappy and withdrew from her colleagues. They, in turn, saw her withdrawal as a rebuke and began to ignore her. The more they avoided her, the more she languished.

By the end of six months, Jackie's languishing and brooding created a self-fulfilling prophecy; because she had fallen behind her deadlines, her new projects were assigned to someone else, hence placing her job in serious jeopardy.

The plain and simple truth is people dislike and avoid feedback because they believe they're being criticized. To clarify, criticism has its place. Professor and thought-leader Adam Grant adds, "People are remarkably open to criticism when they believe it's intended to help them."

Psychiatrist and human resources consultant Jay Jackman theorized that the reason people are so sensitive to hearing about their weaknesses is that they associate feedback with the critical comments received in *childhood* from parents and teachers. Regrettably, fears and assumptions about feedback often show up as psychologically unconscious behaviors, such as procrastination, denial, brooding, jealousy, and self-sabotage.[14]

Embracing a *Lead2Flourish* mindset is vital for your wellbeing. You can adapt to feedback and free yourself from these usual tendencies. You can learn to acknowledge negative emotions, constructively reframe fear and criticism, develop realistic goals, create support systems, and reward yourself for achievements—all hallmarks of flourishing.

Here's how Adam Grant refers to feedback and asking for help:

"Requesting feedback doesn't signal insecurity. It demonstrates that you care more about your learning than your ego. Seeking advice doesn't reveal incompetence. It reflects respect for another person's insight. Asking for help doesn't display weakness. It builds strength."

CHAPTER 5: Myths & Misinformation: Recognizing The Damages

How to Recognize Feedback Phobia Behaviors

Feedback can trigger several *fighting-ego* reactions associated with unconscious behaviors, such as:

- **Feeling helpless, anxious, and dissatisfied.** Abrupt changes in your emotional state like these are generally associated with procrastination. Procrastination is usually unconscious and commonly contains an element of hostility or anger.

- **Unwillingness to face reality.** When you fail to acknowledge the implications of the situation, this is a clue that you're in *denial*. Denial is most often an unconscious reaction to feedback.

- **Lapsing into passivity, paralysis, and isolation.** This is a clue that you're stuck in an emotional state of brooding. You may feel that you can't master the situation. You may recognize this clue in Jackie's situation, which we talked about earlier.

- **Over-idealizing others as more competent or talented.** If you're struggling with others' recognition, you're in an unconscious jealousy trap. For example, Carolyn had what I refer to as comparison fever with one of her female colleagues and believed that she could never rise to that level. Her obsession with this notion drove her to lose all enthusiasm for her work. Instead of seeking feedback from her boss, she allowed jealousy to consume her and ultimately quit her job.

- **Undercutting yourself.** Self-sabotage is common among leaders. Let's refer back to Jerry's story in Chapter 3. Remember how he was overheard complaining about not being appreciated because he resented the negative feedback during a meeting? But instead of initiating further discussion with his colleagues about the feedback, Jerry was caught up in his *fighting-ego* cycle that eventually damaged his relationships.

/ LEAD2FLOURISH

Getting better at receiving feedback starts with understanding and managing those behaviors. Keep in mind that recognizing behavior patterns like these requires awareness and practice. Self-awareness is a skill that, like a muscle, needs a good workout to stay strong and flexible. Feedback can be even more powerful and effective when we are aware of our emotions, beliefs, and actions. In most cases, others are very accurate at detecting unconscious communication. Thus, becoming more self-aware can lead to more relational success within an organization.

THREE PRINCIPLES OF UNDOING FEEDBACK PHOBIAS

Psychologist Albert Ellis constructed an effective technique called Cognitive Reframing, with the idea that "it's not about what happens to you but how you frame it." We briefly mentioned this concept earlier. This tool can work well for undoing feedback phobias. With cognitive reframing, we can change the way we look at something, which consequently changes how we experience it. That kind of approach enables us to reconstruct the feedback process to our advantage. Specifically, this involves putting the prospect of asking for or responding to feedback in a positive light, appreciating rather than rejecting it.

Revisiting Jackie's example the feedback stung, and Jackie, unfortunately, interpreted it as hard criticism.

1. Reframe it

In her mind, Jackie heard rejection and disapproval. The meaning of feedback changed, and her thinking and behavior changed along with it. If she had reframed what she heard, she would've received it as what it was: constructive feedback. All it takes is being able to look at a situation from a slightly different perspective.

Here's what Jackie could've done:

Instead of seeing the feedback as painful, Jackie could've possibly used it to modify her presentation skills and further her career. *"They're right; my*

CHAPTER 5: Myths & Misinformation: Recognizing The Damages

presentations aren't very lively. I've always been uncomfortable with public speaking."

2. Reflect on it

After looking at the situation from a different perspective, you can reflect on several essential questions to better shine a light on the matter. Had Jackie done this, her unhelpful and negative reactions could've been avoided.

Here's what Jackie could've done:

Instead of reacting in an immature manner, a more professional and constructive response would be appropriate. *"How essential is this skill to my job? How can I improve? How much do I want to keep this job? How much am I willing to practice my presentation skills?"* Constructive behaviors are more effective for others to model.

3. Restructure it

Turn floundering into flourishing! Remember how Jackie's performance and wellbeing dipped after her bruised ego couldn't accept and process the feedback?

Here's what Jackie could've done:

Instead of brooding, Jackie could've easily restructured her gloomy behavior with theories: (1) *dynamic presentations are indeed critical to success in sales*, (2) *I'm willing to practice my presentation skills*, or (3) *dynamic presentations aren't necessary for me to succeed.*

Here's what you can do to maintain a flourishing mindset when receiving feedback:

- **Find the intention.** Ask the feedbacker to clarify the goal and to see how you can work together to improve your work. Let him or her know you want it to be a two-way dialogue, where both parties can express personal views rather than argue.

not about me... about the work

- **Separate yourself from your work.** Arguably one of the things that make receiving feedback the most difficult is that the feedback is often taken as a personal critique. Let the feedbacker know that your work is being evaluated and not you. You can say something along the lines of "I understand that the feedback you are providing to me today is not personal feedback; it has everything to do about my work and not who I am as a person."

- **Identify internal discomfort.** It's not uncommon to experience feelings like stress or worry about the idea of receiving feedback. Practice observing and accepting this internal discomfort. Take slow, deep breaths before the feedback session to allow your emotions to subside and not interfere. It's important that you come across as calm and composed because emotions are contagious and can spread from you to the feedbacker.

When you set aside snap reactions and explore where feedback is coming from and where it's going, you garner a stronger Lead2Flourish mentality and enter richer conversations and relationships.

Lead2Flourish Keys

1. Receiving and acting on feedback is a vital ingredient to the development of leaders in today's business world.
2. If you want to flourish in leadership and be successful, you need quality feedback.
3. People dislike and avoid feedback because they believe they're being criticized.
4. One psychiatrist theorized that the reason people are so sensitive to hearing about their weaknesses is that they associate feedback with the critical comments received in childhood from parents and teachers.

CHAPTER 5: Myths & Misinformation: Recognizing The Damages

5. The best leaders ask for feedback. Asking for help doesn't display weakness. It builds strength.

Questions for Reflection

1. What triggers my anxiety when receiving feedback?
2. What personal belief am I holding onto that I fear will be revealed in receiving feedback?
3. Which of the five *fighting-ego* responses to feedback have I experienced?
4. Which of the three techniques for reversing feedback phobias work best for me?
5. Which of the three practices works best to maintain a flourishing mindset?

Designing a Lead2Flourish Plan – Challenging the Feedback Myth

Reflecting on what you've learned in this segment, practice defying the defensive, protective mechanism when receiving feedback. Design a plan to enhance your feedback "curiosity" and receive it as a growth tool.

1. The psychological behaviors I'm facing are:
2. I've decided to commit to:
3. The reasons I've made this decision are:
4. Potential *fighting-ego* hurdles:
5. In what ways can I become open to feedback?
6. How will I introduce to my organization the importance of executives receiving and constructively processing feedback and taking action to work on any areas for improvement?
7. My timeline:

BEHAVIOR MYTH #4:
WORK AND LIFE MUST BALANCE

One Life, No Tradeoffs

Work-life balance, as we understand it, often requires that we make tradeoffs, compromising satisfaction in one or more areas of our lives to fulfill our responsibilities in another. Unfortunately, compromising in this way can leave us feeling inauthentic, disconnected, and stressed.[15]

Meet Natalie

Appearances can be misleading. To her friends, Natalie seemed to live her best life. As a talented forty-four-year-old vice president of a public relations firm, many would say she had it all: a challenging and promising career, a supportive spouse, two wonderful children, a beautiful suburban home, and a seat on the board of an advertising company. Natalie's days were full and busy. Getting to the gym at 4:30 a.m. before her children woke up, then getting back home in time to eat breakfast with them before heading out to work. Evenings, she returned home just before the children's bedtime. The next day she did it all again.

On the surface, Natalie seemed to be doing great, but the truth is, she was falling apart on the inside. She barely held things together and was borderline burned out. Feeling exhausted and overwhelmed, Natalie decided to confide in her friend Suzanne about the little spats between her and her husband. He'd complained about feeling neglected.

Natalie told Suzanne that she didn't feel in charge of her life and didn't seem to be succeeding in any one area. With spending so much time at work, Natalie was stressed over fulfilling the rest of her responsibilities. Finding a balance between her work and life was the goal. That's when Suzanne suggested that she talk with us to learn what a flourishing life might look like for her.

CHAPTER 5: Myths & Misinformation: Recognizing The Damages

Work is not the opposite of life. Work and life are interrelated domains constantly presented separately, competing for time and energy.

Where Did Work-Life Balance Come From?

The notion that one should limit the amount of time spent at work dates back to manufacturing laws of the late 1800s when the work hours of women and children were restricted. The first move to give workers back more time occurred on October 24, 1940, when the US officially amended the Fair Labor Standards Act and adopted the forty-hour work week.[16] The description "work-and-life balance" was born, as Tom Brown put it, in *Industry Week Magazine* in 1986:

> **"A Minneapolis consultant and author, Dick Leider paints a picture of managers struggling to capture a mythical thing called "balance"—a proportioning of their lives with sufficient weight on professional activities, but with a healthy counterweight of family and personal interests. 'It used to be that work-and-life balance was a boutique issue,' he says."**

Brown used the description again in 1988 but dropped the word 'and,' referring to it as we know it today: "work-life balance."

Unraveling the Myth

The concept of balance refers to equilibrium or evenness. Then, if life includes work (and it does), and work is a part of life (and it is), how can work and life be even? It's not a science. Think about what "work" includes for leaders: managing, operating, paperwork, administrative duties, teaching, committee work, coaching, presentations, traveling, conferences, meetings, etc.

Life is generally everything else. Now think about what "life" is for a leader: commitment to family, friends, and community; physical needs, such as exercise, nutrition, personal health, and sleep; activities that promote spiritual and emotional wellbeing, and activities of daily living, such as laundry, paying bills, and performing household chores. Here's an interesting fact: a leader's responsibilities aren't restricted to physical hours spent at work and can spill over onto life hours as well.

Looking at the various elements that comprise "work" and "life," it becomes immediately clear why the idea that we can have a "work-life balance" is indeed a myth.

No On and Off Switch

Natalie faced a hard challenge. Not only did her responsibilities interfere with quality time spent with her family, but she was also harming her wellbeing. This is where the fighting-ego insidiously slips in. As we do more, we unconsciously see it as a way to acquire more power. And with that, we feel the need to do even more with the time that we have. It's tempting to push ourselves to perform for recognition. We already know how this pleases the ego and how attention makes us feel. We saw that earlier with Travis, who went to any length to prove that he was an achiever. What I discovered from my own experience and the research is that finding equilibrium and evenness in work, family, relationships, community service, and self-time isn't doable. We don't have the capacity to switch from work to life management. There's no on and off switch given at birth.

But synchronizing these different life endeavors can be achieved. This is a holistic approach to living that enables people to create wins across varying life domains. So, we asked Natalie this question: Wouldn't it be more convenient and fulfilling to forget about trying to balance what's not balanceable and instead process work in the same way you perform life? Yes,

CHAPTER 5: Myths & Misinformation: Recognizing The Damages

she agreed! We showed her the way to integrate and transition work and life seamlessly as she realigned priorities by what she loved.

Think about it. When priorities drive our lives, we make the most out of every day. This enthusiasm and energy is called zest—the capacity to feel revved up and ready to go.

There's even early research to show us why this matters. A 2009 article in the *Journal of Organizational Behavior* detailed three separate studies on the impact of having zest in work and life. The sample consisted of 9,803 employed adult respondents from six occupational groups. The first study measured strength-relevant statements about themselves. The second study measured respondents' stances toward work and life. The third measured respondents' evaluation of satisfaction with life in general.

The studies concluded that zest is a primarily important factor for work and general life satisfaction and an overall sense of self. Zest, also known as a heart strength, is a trait of gratitude, hope, and love and predicts a person's happiness and level of contentment in his or her work and personal life.[17]

Realigning our priorities (another way of looking on the bright side of things) helps us to feel lively and high-spirited every day. This conditions our brains to form neural networks that make us feel joyful, which is why zestful leaders don't have to put in much effort to extract positivity—you reflect it spontaneously.

The University of Michigan study found that the urge to learn new things and apply them to the workplace is a great stressbuster, and people who did something active, such as engaging themselves in learning, were twice as happy and satisfied with their jobs than people who participated in passive activities. Again, this trait, which scientists closely related to zest, guaranteed better integration of work and life and increased productivity.[18]

LEAD2FLOURISH

SIX PRINCIPLES OF INTEGRATING WORK AND LIFE

Zest can be an important barometer for integrating work and life. Writer Paulo Coelho said, "When you are enthusiastic about what you do, you feel the positive energy." This enthusiasm and energy create zest. Practice these principles to help you boost your zest so you can seamlessly integrate work and life.

1. Recognize zest zappers

Psychologist and professor Martin Seligman's studies on zest concluded its importance in work and life because of its link to psychological wellbeing. As well as being a key element in integrating work and life, did you know that zest depletes itself as we perform tasks grudgingly, focusing more on the negative aspects of life and surrendering during times of distress?

Here's what you need to know:

Sometimes we unconsciously loosen our grip on a zestful lifestyle as we fall into routine traps and habits. The list below shows a lifestyle that zaps our zest over time:

- Distracting habits
- Rushing around
- Feeling inadequate
- Working endless hours
- Overloading on information
- Using time unwisely
- Demanding tasks
- Existing, not living
- Doing what you don't enjoy
- Lacking sufficient downtime

2. Kick your zest into gear

Bob Proctor said, "In times of unrest and in an unstable economy, it's very easy to let your attitude slip and begin feeling sorry for yourself. This is precisely when you want to practice healthy attitudinal rules to stay alert, alive, and enthusiastic. Don't ever lose the zest for life, and life won't lose its zest for you. Say something positive to every person you meet today."

Here's what you can do:

Practice this simple technique to re-energize and build your zest. Draw a grid with four quadrants and label them as shown below. Fill in activities that belong in each square or section, and then assign percentages to each. You'll realize that you're spending far too much time doing activities that drain your energy, both at home and at work. Gradually increase the amount of time you spend on activities that build energy.[19]

Builds my energy at home	% time spent here	Drains my energy at home	% time spent here
Builds my enery at work	% time spent here	Drains my energy at work	% time spent here

3. *Eliminate the competition mindset*

If you're thinking of ways to get work done and then ways of getting life done, your mind has work and life in competition. Stop competing with yourself. It's all your life. This behavior only leads to exhaustion and burnout.

LEAD2FLOURISH

Here's what you can do:

See every activity in your day as a part of a whole. Your goal is to visualize work and life roles as being interconnected and dependent on each other, rather than separate and competing for your time and energy.

4. Batch it

Batching is a productivity method in which similar tasks are grouped and executed in one swoop. It eliminates the decision fatigue of trying to fit in all your daily activities.

Here's what you need to do:

Instead of responding to every email as it comes in, set a time to review them all in one batch. Combine both family-related and work-related errands in one batch. When possible, designate two or three days a week for both external meetings and video conference calls. You can also maintain your zest and get more of your time and energy back by batching and reserving meetings for specific days.

5. Maintain firm boundaries

Honor yourself and your commitments to maintaining zest and synchronizing the important areas of life.

Here's what you need to do:

Don't apologize for building a wall around the activities that drain your energy, both at home and at work. If an emergency meeting springs up during your personal time, repay yourself by replacing that time later on. This could mean setting aside blocks of time on weekends for focused work and blocks of time on weekdays for personal activities.

6. Commit to a flourishing attitude

By being real (acting authentically), whole (acting with integrity), and innovative (acting with creativity), you can integrate all life domains. This empowers you to maintain a flourishing attitude. Not only does it serve you well in your efforts to be a better leader, but this combination also helps you to enhance your performance wellbeing.

Here's what you need to do:

Think about the actions you can take and what's in your power that will add value, bring harmony, and improve outcomes in every life domain: work, family, relationships, community service, and self-time.

Lead2Flourish Keys

1. Researchers theorized that the stress of having to decide between work and home showed drops in creativity and higher levels of cognitive dissonance.
2. An obsession with "balancing" events and interactions in your life could lead to losing your spontaneity—simply going through the motions of life instead of truly living life.
3. Instead of thinking of work and life as equals, make life your priority and acknowledge that what you do for work is simply a part of that life.
4. Synchronizing is a holistic approach to living that enables people to create wins across varying life domains.
5. When priorities drive our lives, we make the most out of every day. This enthusiasm and energy is called zest—the capacity to feel revved up and ready to go.
6. Scientists associated zest as a trait for the integration of work and life and increased productivity.
7. Studies concluded that zest is a primarily important factor for work and general life satisfaction and an overall sense of self.

Questions for Reflection

1. Thinking about how life includes work and work is a part of life, how can work and life balance and be even?
2. If work-life balance, as we've been taught, often requires that we make tradeoffs, is it possible to make tradeoffs among work, family, community, and self?
3. What does integrating work and life mean for me?
4. How will I synchronize life and work to have more time for creative projects and personal time with less anxiety?

Designing a Lead2Flourish Plan – Undoing Work-Life Balance Behavior

Reflecting on what you've learned in this segment, knowing that work-life balance isn't a tug-of-war, design a plan that includes work for what it is—a part of life.

1. The behaviors I need to adopt that will serve me well are:
2. I'm committing to this specific vision of work-life integration:
3. I'm committed to this decision because:
4. Potential *fighting-ego* hurdles:
5. I can maximize what I love about life and work by:
6. I will introduce the work-life balance myth to my organization by:
7. My timeline:

STAGE 2

RENOVATING

Sometimes we must tear down the old to build the new. In this stage, we'll renovate dysfunctional, destructive behaviors that interfere with your true essence, expressed in the consistency between your vision, values, and voice and deconstruct behavior myths that undermine your progress. This design stage helps with aligning ethical decision-making, workplace demands, and cultivating a genuine connection with people and work.

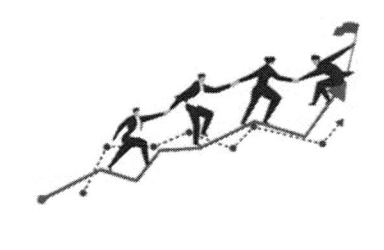

CHAPTER 6

RENOVATING TO REALIZE VALUES: THE GUIDING FOUNDATION

―

Personal Journey to Realizing Values

Having and holding to a core set of values is an essential part of flourishing. It gives you purpose, direction, and motivation. I shamefully admit that when I worked in corporate leadership, I didn't hold myself or my team to a core set of personal values. Ouch! The truth is, I was caught up in performing to look good. Not purpose, but more selfish behavior. Professor Adam Grant said, "Meaningful work isn't about impressing others. It's about expressing your values."

Now I see this was one of the biggest mistakes I made in my professional journey. Ignoring the importance of personal values and interpreting your values in alignment with those of the organization is an oversight no leader should ever make.

It's not that I didn't know what I valued. We all do to a certain degree. Writing it down and expressing it in ways to inspire others is what I neglected to do. I thought I'd placed a high value on people's growth and development, but my values were out of line. Perhaps I became relaxed because I knew that I could count on people in key positions to get the job done, especially a smart lady named Yvonne. She was my go-to girl for sniffing out those problematic areas, which freed me to focus on more important things, you know, what we call the leadership stuff.

My department stayed on top of the game and excelled when other departments didn't. I was proud of that. Then out of the blue, my senior vice president snatched (at least that's how I saw it) Yvonne from my department and transferred her to help another area get up to speed. Yvonne seemed empowered by this new opportunity, and it was apparent that she was hungry for more challenges. But I was devastated. She was a key player that I didn't want or expect to lose. While taking this transfer as a personal attack, my childhood insecurities resurfaced and triggered behaviors that created and enforced silos. It became noticeably obvious that I didn't want to interact effectively and efficiently with the other department. Today I can see how my *fighting-ego* blindsided me. No leader can flourish this way.

Ignoring the overarching corporate goals and neglecting my values caused me to base my loyalty on my department and not on the company as a whole. Had I created a culture of values, I would've been driven by them and gladly released Yvonne with my blessings instead of pouting and counting my losses. Realizing the embarrassment caused by my ego-driven reactions to Yvonne's transfer motivated me to renovate my selfish behavioral tendencies. Reframing the situation enabled me to shift my mindset toward a different perspective and accept Yvonne's transfer as good for the whole company.

CHAPTER 6: Renovating To Realize Values: The Guiding Foundation

Why Renovate to Realize Values

Steve Jobs once said, "The only thing that works is management by values."[1] Values are powerful drivers of how we think and behave. Realizing values is a repetitive behavior that's necessary to *Lead2Flourish*.

Values are tied in with ethics and morals. They offer us a reliable and guiding foundation that we can use to guide our judgment and choose our actions. Values heighten our self-realization. Our character, whether in or out of the office, is expressed by our values. Whether we're at work or home, values don't change. Values are at the heart of what we stand for. They're unique and individualized. We all choose different combinations of values in life, and these choices shape our life decisions. As leaders, realizing our values helps us to prioritize our professional goals and understand what we truly want to become. Renovating, as I did, to realize values is the pathway to leading from our highest selves.

We Are the Behaviors Others See

Being our personal best as leaders includes exhibiting behaviors in line with both core values and ethics. As a former corporate leader, I can assure you that we live them in our actions every single day. Values are the vehicles that transport how we think and what we say, which ultimately directs our behavior. Our behavior is the ultimate expression of what we value. We are the behaviors others see.

Psychologists also believe in the transformative power of values. Their studies show that ethics and values can change our inner world and alter the way we perceive and react to stimuli.[2] Here are three key ways this works:

1. A leader who has regard for honesty will genuinely reflect this behavior by their actions. He or she is less likely to engage in behaviors such as lying, stealing, cheating, or using any unfair means to accomplish his or her goals.

LEAD2FLOURISH

2. Leaders who value personal integrity are less likely to make decisions know to be injurious to someone else.
3. Leaders who say he or she values an idea recognize that their behaviors must back it up.

Oftentimes, what leaders say and what they do aren't congruent. If that happens, others assume they are untrustworthy and, therefore, will not follow them.

If I asked you to explain why you do what you do, you could probably rattle off a few things. But if I ask you if people can see your authentic values in what you do, now that might stump you. Why is that? Values are developed as we grow. At times, we don't understand what's most important to us. Instead, we focus on the conventional values of our society, culture, and the media. When it comes to working, we tend to adopt the values we were taught to follow. In the political landscape, we tend to accept the values of our party of choice.

However, when we are truly ethical and principled, we believe in our values to the point where they are an integral and subconscious part of our person. Being principled is a very powerful method of influence. A strong set of values can have a good return on investment (ROI). And once we memorialize our own deep personal values on paper, then our lives and our leadership take on a whole new meaning.

Discovering what drives you or your values is important, but identifying what drives you as a leader is what will take you to the next level and enable you to flourish. Operating with a *Lead2Flourish* mindset is identifying your authentic values, not simply emulating other leaders or key figures in your industry, and knowing these are behind the purpose of all your decisions.

Answer These Questions

I want you to take some time to think about the following questions to help you discover your deepest-held core beliefs.

CHAPTER 6: Renovating To Realize Values: The Guiding Foundation

1. How do you want others to experience you?
2. How often do you participate in self-evaluation?
3. Do you know how your beliefs affect your decisions?
4. How would your colleagues describe you?
5. What is the inner motor that pushes you to get to the heart of an issue and find solutions?
6. What drives your behavior and guides the choices you make in your daily life?

FIVE PRINCIPLES OF VALUE-DRIVEN BEHAVIOR

At the core of a leader's psychological wellbeing is value-based leadership. A leader's values and how those values impact others day-by-day are fundamental for being our best. Values are the GPS for the way we do everything. Values are the life force of how we lead, a permanent platform to stand on that allows us to make decisions from a place of conviction. From my studies on effective leaders, I would say there are five value-driven personalities that enable flourishing outcomes.

1. Genuinely self-confident

As playwright and poet E.E. Cummings said, "Once we believe in ourselves, we can risk curiosity, wonder, spontaneous delight, or any experience that reveals the human spirit." It is a bold step to accept ourselves as we are. Given that we recognize our strengths, we must also recognize our weaknesses. With true self-confidence, we acknowledge our accomplishments and expertise while recognizing there will always be someone more accomplished and successful. Knowing this, we can own our value. For example, if you value success and status and fall short or make a mistake, you won't beat up on yourself or feel condemned. You confidently and unashamedly strive for continuous improvement.

Here's what you need to know:

Self-confidence creates the platform for better decision-making, a clearer self-image, and constructive behavior. We can make decisions faster and be more confident when we know and understand what's most important to us. We can also understand if our values are undermining our self-image and, when necessary, build beliefs and behaviors to replace them. We can connect with people and organizations that are in alignment with those values and adjust where they don't.

2. *Genuinely self-reflective*

Research has shown that we think more than 50,000 thoughts per day, of which more than half are negative, and more than 90% are just repeated from the day before.[3] Making time to refocus the mind on positivity through self-reflection allows us to discover what we deem important. Learning more about our values helps us to take power away from distractions and refocus on fulfillment. Self-reflection is not devolving into "woe is me" thinking. It's seeking to understand those innate characteristics that have been providentially put in our DNA. In times of reflection, you'll unearth your core values, the things that you care about deeply that empower you to confidently live a credible and compelling life full of purpose in your style and manner.

Here's what you need to do:

Practice reflecting on what you stand for and what matters most to you. I find it amusing to observe leaders who think that their values are obvious to them, but they have no idea at all. Understand the importance of living and contributing your values without scrambling to recall the corporate values. Often, we develop our most important values unconsciously. Self-reflection brings them into consciousness. In other words, know thyself. And because your values are the why behind your behaviors, time spent in self-reflection will greatly equip you to maintain an effective leadership presence.

CHAPTER 6: Renovating To Realize Values: The Guiding Foundation

3. Genuinely psychologically open

How often do you look at situations from multiple perspectives and different viewpoints to gain a much fuller understanding of things? We talked about this in a previous chapter. I haven't yet met a leader who admits to being psychologically closed and afraid to test their ideas with others. However, most leaders that I've worked with were somewhat secretive and emotionally distant from their employees and didn't see the need to bounce ideas off them, or they disliked it when their beliefs were challenged.

No doubt, as leaders, we face compromising situations. But having a system of personal values in place makes navigating these circumstances much easier. For example, if you value teamwork, your psychological openness removes the anxiety and uncertainty of considering different views and opinions. A willingness to allow ourselves to be influenced by other people and to share our ideas openly enhances the know-how. With awareness of what we value as a leader, psychological openness celebrates diverse perspectives.

Here's what you need to do:

Discipline yourself to share your values and expectations with your subordinates. Start observing how collaborative perspectives help with innovation and creative problem-solving.

4. Genuinely humble

I believe that the most misunderstood principle of value-based leadership is humility—the quality of being modest and humble. The truth is that we cannot lead from our highest selves if we feel we are better and more important than our subordinates. Others may report directly to us, but we must never forget who we are and where we came from. For this reason, our personal values help us to stay grounded in the humanity within each of us.

For example, poor decisions are made when we place too much trust in our judgment. When our core values include contribution and community, we can easily acknowledge our limitations and vulnerabilities and seek the advice of others. Genuine humility also helps us value each person we encounter and treat everyone with respect. It's about renovating to recognize and accept the humanity within each of us.

Here's what you need to do:

Be open to helping others perform their jobs better. Offer your help as their equal, not as their boss. Encourage your employees to share their voices and demonstrate respect for their knowledge, skills, creativity, and entrepreneurial spirit.

5. *A genuine realist*

I like how realism was explained by inspirational writer William Arthur Ward: "The pessimist complains about the wind; the optimist expects it to change; the realist adjusts the sails." I believe Ward was saying, instead of letting your *fighting-ego* take the driver's seat, the realist weighs in and evaluates information to determine the best direction to take. The realistic leader knows when to finetune, correct, and make necessary changes, which may require a willingness to interact with colleagues, customers, or employees to adjust the sails. I haven't met many leaders who are willing to sit back and receive the hand reality deals them, but it's a valuable ability.

Questions for Reflection – Realizing Values

It's time to increase awareness of what matters to you by identifying your top five values that can make a genuine difference in your life and your leadership. Questions to keep in mind are: *What's important to me in my life? What do I enjoy doing? When do I feel satisfied and fulfilled?* Awareness of your values moves you toward the behaviors that are in line with them.

1. Take time to reflect on your values. My values are:
2. Prioritize your values and select five of your most important ones. My

CHAPTER 6: Renovating To Realize Values: The Guiding Foundation

    top five values are:

3. Take a deep breath and meditate on what each of these values means to you. Then, come up with a definition that resonates and makes sense to you.

Value *a* means to me:	Is important to me because:
Value *b* means to me:	Is important to me because:
Value *c* means to me:	Is important to me because:
Value *d* means to me:	Is important to me because:
Value *e* means to me:	Is important to me because:

4. Reflect on how your actions have been consistent or inconsistent with these values.
5. What behavior would you need to look for that would prove that you are living out these values?

Lead2Flourish Keys

1. The only thing that works is management by values.
2. Your behavior is the ultimate expression of what you value.
3. You are the behaviors others see.
4. When we memorialize our own deep personal values on paper, then our lives and our leadership take on a whole new meaning.
5. Discovering what drives you as a leader is what enables flourishing.
6. Operating with a *Lead2Flourish* mindset is identifying your authentic values and knowing these are behind the purpose of all your decisions.

Designing a Lead2Flourish Plan – Renovating to Realize Values

Reflecting on what you've learned in this chapter on the importance of personal values and translating them into the mission of the organization, design a plan that renovates behaviors that don't align with whom you want to be, so you can include your values in this mission.

1. I am now motivated to renovate these behavioral areas:
2. The behaviors I need to adopt that will serve me well are:
3. The reasons I've made this decision are:
4. Potential *fighting-ego* hurdles:
5. I use values to guide my judgment and prepare me to choose my actions by:
6. This is how I will introduce the importance of realizing values to my organization:
7. My timeline:

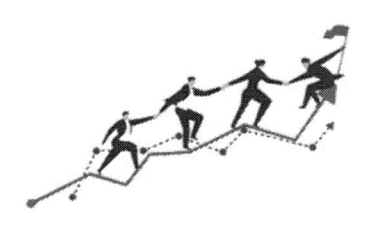

CHAPTER 7

RENOVATING TO REALIZE VISION: WHAT YOU EXPECT TO SEE

The Man in the Park

I read a story about a man who sat motionless on an amusement park bench, mesmerized as he stared into space. He was being watched by a maintenance worker who thought it was very strange behavior. With curiosity, the maintenance worker asked, "How are you, sir?" Without looking at the maintenance worker, the man said, "Fine," and kept staring intently into space. Then the worker said, "Sir, what are you doing?" "I'm looking at my mountain," the man responded. "I see my mountain right there."

Absorbed in his imaginary concept of a futuristic space mountain, the man rushed to describe it to his architects to draw the plans exactly as he'd dreamed.

But unfortunately, the man died before the mountain was constructed. The man's name was Walt Disney. Still, Mr. Disney's Space Mountain was eventually built and today accommodates several thrill rides. At its dedication ceremony, Mrs. Disney was present, along with the mayor and governor.

As the ceremony began, the young man who introduced Mrs. Disney asserted, "It's a pity that Mr. Disney is not here today to see this mountain, but we're glad his wife is here." Mrs. Disney walked up to the podium, looked at the crowd, and said, in effect, "I must correct this young man. Walt already saw the mountain. It is you who are just now seeing it."[1] Every year, thousands of people visit this Space Mountain in Magic Kingdom Park at Walt Disney World Resort.

To See or Not to See

As we take on leadership roles, often what is seen are the mountains we want to be moved out of our way. We don't take time to stare into the unseen. We don't see which course to take or what lies ahead. We don't create timeouts to reassess our lives and strategies and focus on our vision. We instead follow through on behaviors that cause us to make the same mistakes and decisions that have hijacked us in the past.

What this means is that we tend to depend on the neurochemical system that regulates thoughts and emotions at the moment to help us navigate the complexities of life. Taking time to see further than we can look, with the ability to articulate it in a way that's both compelling and inclusive, escapes us. These are personal structural issues in need of renovation.

A Harvard Business Review article noted that less than 20% of leaders have a strong sense of individual purpose.[2] These same leaders can articulate the vision of the company but fail to provide clarity on how they plan to fit their vision into the whole system. It doesn't matter if you're the CEO of a multi-million-dollar company or leading a small team of three; your purpose is what makes you who you are. It's your why: why you're working, why you

CHAPTER 7: Renovating To Realize Vision: What You Expect To See

want to lead the team, and more. That's the difference between being a leader and being an effective leader. Like Walt Disney, the latter has a future in mind. This is the reason some leaders get remembered and acknowledged long after they're gone.

Start With Why

Unfortunately, because of our behavior tendencies, we lean toward the *what* and *how* in getting things done while skipping over the *why*. Knowing why your role is important, committing to your *why*—or your vision—and values that highlight your ideal behavior will reveal your true purpose as a leader.

In his book, *Start with Why: How Great Leaders Inspire Action*, Simon Sinek's *why* is grounded in the tenets of the biology of human decision-making. He expounds on what he calls *The Golden Circle*—a diagram that works perfectly with how our brain works. The circle comprises three outward concentric circles with the inner circle as the *why*, the next layer as the *how,* and the outer layer defined by the *what*.

Sinek explains that the outer section of the Golden Circle—the *what*—corresponds to the outer section of the brain: the neocortex. This part of the brain is responsible for rational and analytical thought. It helps us understand facts and figures, features, and benefits. The why and how are the middle two sections

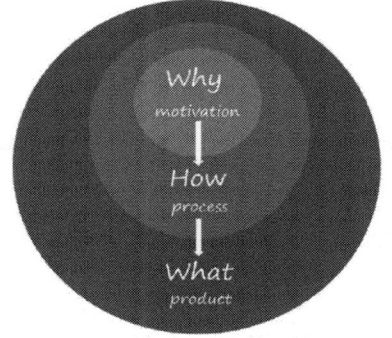

Inspired by Simon Sinek's Golden Circle Theory

of the Golden Circle that correspond to the middle section of the brain, the limbic system. This part of the brain is responsible for our behavior, decision-making, and emotions, like trust and loyalty. Sinek contends that leaders and teams know what they do, and how they do it, but very few can articulate *why* they do what they do.

It's not so surprising then to see a company's vision carried out and supported by diverse input from the individual visions of its leaders. That is, one department may go in one direction and another department can take a different course, yet still come together at fulfilling the vision of the company. However, if companies are to establish a firm commitment to its business values and vision, their leader must likewise be able to grasp, articulate, and blend their individual values and vision instead of acting on their gut feelings.

Why We Struggle With "Why"

As Viktor Frankl described in his 1946 book, *Man's Search for Meaning*, he survived the Holocaust and three years of incarceration in Nazi concentration camps. Frankl, in addition, demonstrated many critical visionary skills throughout his experience. He understood the importance of values in life, had a strong awareness of his own, and lived by them. In doing so, he found his meaning and purpose. He exhibited constructive thought strategies and continuously identified opportunities to contribute to the wellbeing of his inmates. His visionary skills helped him to persevere in this way, not only throughout the entire period of incarceration but afterward too.[3]

It seems safe and appropriate then to use *why, vision,* and *meaning* interchangeably. Frankl learned a valuable lesson about vision in an unexpected way. He believed that humans have both freedom and responsibility to bring forth their best possible selves by realizing the meaning of the moment in every situation—in other words, their *why, vision* and *purpose*. But it's interesting to note how leaders struggle with this. Why is it that leaders can easily communicate the *what* and the *how* of the whole system but struggle with communicating their personal *why*? Behaviors learned from a childhood event could be the reason. Let's examine three possibilities from the experiences of Tim, Ricky, and Michael.

CHAPTER 7: Renovating To Realize Vision: What You Expect To See

Limited Options

When his team zeroed in on a few options to take them out of a dilemma, Tim rejected the possibility of any of them working. Instead of going along with the strategic opportunity, he naturally succumbed to his *fighting-ego*. From early childhood, Tim was conditioned to make decisions based only on what he could see. Searching beyond what was in front of him wasn't his approach to life or work. In his mind, if it wasn't before him, it didn't exist, which limited his range of options. As a habit, choices were founded on this learned principle. Tim was uncomfortable strengthening his connection to his *why* and drawing from an infinite range of possibilities that made having a personal vision almost impossible.

Limited Resources

Ricky was asked to observe and document the behavior and performance of an executive team to be used as a learning tool and visionary guide for new hires. Ricky became visibly uncomfortable with this. Growing up, Ricky loved imagining himself in the roles of his superheroes. He abruptly stopped all forms of visualizing after his parents told him it was unnatural to imagine himself as an action figure. His parents often scolded him for pretending to be a superhero. From that incident, Ricky's paranoia led him to give up the whole idea of visualization, believing that envisioning the future carried no benefits. He often suggested to his team that there was no need to expand on what was already working for them. Ricky wasn't aware that the more he visualized, the better he would get at developing this skill and creating the future of his team from his imagination.

Limited Reality

Michael's employees weren't inspired by his leadership style mainly because he wanted everything to be perfect. This placed unnecessary strain on their relationships. As far back as he could remember, Michael had been compelled to be a perfectionist. The perfectionist in him needed to craft a timeless and ideal vision statement. He believed his vision had to be exactly right and feared that if the project failed, it would reflect poorly on his competence. Naturally, this wasn't realistic.

Renovating to Realizing Vision

The late Dr. Myles Munroe stated that "to have vision means to see something coming into view as if it were already there."[4] This means having a dream or destination in mind, not relating by any means to the law of attraction. Realizing vision, articulating and demonstrating it to others certainly penetrates the essence of our *why*, doesn't it? However, before we can share our vision with others, we first need to realize our *why*. Seems easy enough, right? Often, it's not. We all like to think we know why we're leaders, but deeply searching out what's in our hearts, seeing it coming into view as if it were already there, and articulating it with passion can be challenging.

Unfortunately, many of us leaders allow our *fighting-ego* to dodge the necessary work. But in the process of realizing a vision, we must first renovate unhelpful behaviors to discover how to take our why from an initial idea to fulfillment. Realizing your *why* enables you to:

- Sense what drives your behavior when you're performing at your best
- Articulate and express what makes you feel fulfilled
- See past obstacles and how to move forward with purpose
- Inspire others to appreciate and join with your vision

Vision Requires Purposeful, Driven Behavior

The late purposive behaviorist Edward Tolman defined purpose quite simply as persistence in behavior. Behavior that has a particular and recognized goal in mind that will aid in achieving that goal. *Purposeful*

CHAPTER 7: Renovating To Realize Vision: What You Expect To See

behavior starts with a commitment to a vision. The goal of the behavior must be derived from an inner vision aimed at benefiting others. That's what makes it purposeful. We must answer the question, "How will others benefit if I achieve this vision?" For example, ask any fan of the late Walt Disney, and they can probably tell you the first time they ever rode the iconic ride at Space Mountain.

Purposeful behavior answers the "why" question that can otherwise place doubts in our minds. Any leader with a personal vision must use focused behavior to effectively navigate to success. And to do this, we need to leave our comfort zone. That's a huge renovation effort in itself. Intentionally leaving the comfort zone goes together with developing a growth mindset. On the other hand, as we saw with the experiences of Tim, Ricky, and Michael, a fixed mindset keeps us trapped by fear of failure. The growth mindset expands what's possible. It inspires us to learn and take healthy risks, leading to positive outcomes across life domains.

Realizing Purposeful Behavior With Visualization

The high-performance core of a leader is where vision is free to develop and expand. In his book, *The Art of Leading by Looking Ahead*, business consultant Rob-Jan de Jong writes, "You have to look beyond the obvious to what stretches the imagination without being absurd. A potent personal vision is imaginative, directed, and often breaks paradigms. And it has the power to mobilize the people around you."[5]

Retired professional golfer Jack Nicklaus asserts, "I never hit a shot, not even in practice, without having a very sharp, in-focus picture of it in my head. First, I see the ball where I want it to finish, nice and white, sitting up high on the bright green grass. Then the scene quickly changes, and I see the ball going there, its path, trajectory, shape, and even its behavior on landing. Then there's a short fade-out, and the next scene shows me making the kind of swing that will turn the previous images into reality."[6]

Nicklaus, widely considered to be one of the greatest golfers of all time, has won 117 professional tournaments in his career. Over a quarter-century, he won a record eighteen major championships and has been named Golfer of the Century by almost every major golf publication in the world. According to him, all his performances and successes are attributed to visualization. It presents the big-picture view that provides direction for the future.

For example, one of my clients, Kim, someone I respected as a highly effective leader, had great communication skills but wasn't inspired by her work. Kim realized she couldn't be a more effective and persuasive leader by only sharpening her presentation skills; she had to define who she was as an individual and what was important to her. After some concentrated dialogue to uncover what was going on in her heart, mind, body, and spirit, she began to connect with her natural creativity and resourcefulness. She started realizing her desired purposeful behavior with visualization. And so can you.

The body reacts to images in the brain as though they are real opportunities. As visualization helps you "rewire" your connections, it ultimately changes your habits. Mental practice is an effective means of enhancing performance, as concluded in the research of psychologists James Driskell, Carolyn Copper, and Aidan Moran.[7]

TWO PRINCIPLES OF REALIZING YOUR PERSONAL VISION

1. A written vision statement serves as your template of purpose.

From the Bible we know that Habakkuk was told to write the vision and clearly inscribe it on tablets, so one may easily read it.[8] A written vision statement serves as your template of purpose. It can be used to introduce, evaluate, and refine, as needed, the purposeful desired behavior. Not only was Habakkuk instructed to write the vision but also to wait for its appointed time to manifest. In other words, to be patient but steady. God knew that visionary leaders would lose interest when reality doesn't appear right away. He knew

CHAPTER 7: Renovating To Realize Vision: What You Expect To See

that the *fighting-ego* couldn't stand failure, weakness, and incompetence, so he directed Habakkuk to wait for it, even if it took a while, and still assured him of its coming.

Here's what you need to do:

Without a vision statement, you run the risk of always putting out fires and paying attention to the pressures of the immediate and sacrificing the future—*what* and *how*. Kim transferred her visualized images—her *why*—into a written vision statement that she could easily read and understand. So can you:

- Combine what you see in your leadership role into an expression of your vision.
- Refine your vision until it expresses exactly what you want it to say.
- Be crystal clear.
- Be as specific as possible.
- Keep it short enough to be memorable, about two to three sentences, for example: We believe that leadership should be fulfilling and rewarding. It should bring you pleasure and gratification. We also believe that every leader can flourish.

2. Align your vision with the organization's

Today, companies understand that corporate visions and personal visions work well together. Why? Because your company needs you to serve its vision in a way that's authentic to you. As you leverage what inspires you in support of your company's mission, you're more dedicated to serving in your best capacity, which ultimately serves the people you work with as well.

Here's what you need to do:

Kim wanted her company to benefit from the unique passions, strengths, and ideas she could contribute. With some soul searching, she aligned her vision as a leader with the vision and mission of the company. You can always find some way to align your vision with that of a company if you try hard enough, unless there's an underlying conflict. In that case, you may need to consider a career change. Begin here:

- Find language that will motivate and energize your team.
- Include your team's values. You're in this together.
- Include the vision of your organization.
- Focus on your uniqueness as a person and on your organization's uniqueness to specify how your values will help you as a leader.
- Emphasize the collective identity of your organization by using words like "we" and "our" and by focusing on what everyone in the organization has in common.

Lead2Flourish Keys

1. Committing to your *why*—or your vision—and values that highlight your ideal behavior to yourself and others reveals your true purpose as a leader.
2. If a company is to establish a firm commitment to its values and vision, its leader must be able to grasp, articulate, and blend her or his values and vision instead of acting on gut feelings.
3. Before we can share our vision with others, we first need to realize our *why*.
4. A written vision statement serves as a template of purpose. It can be used to introduce, evaluate, and refine, as needed, the purposeful behavior required to see its fulfillment.
5. As you leverage what inspires you in support of your company's mission, you're more dedicated to serving in your best capacity that ultimately serves the people you work with as well.

CHAPTER 7: Renovating To Realize Vision: What You Expect To See

Questions for Reflection

To help bring more clarity, use the following questions to visualize what's important to you.

1. What specifically is your *why*?
2. What matters most in your leadership role?
3. What story(s) of achievement would you like to be able to tell in the future?
4. Imagine what it will be like to accomplish these goals. How does it make you feel?
5. What are some positive and concrete images that convey where you want to be?
6. Which images express strength, achievement, collaboration, and influence?
7. What values and challenges are implicit in your goals?
8. What do you and your team value the most about your goals?
9. What kind of person do you need to become, and what behaviors must you uphold to achieve your goals?

Designing a Lead2Flourish Plan – Renovating to Realize Vision

Reflecting on what you've learned in this chapter on the importance of a personal vision fitting into the whole system, design a plan that includes incorporating your vision with the company's vision.

1. The positive behaviors I need to adopt that will serve my *"why"* are:
2. I've decided to commit to:
3. The reasons I've made this decision are:
4. Potential *fighting-ego* hurdles:

LEAD2FLOURISH

5. I will use my "*why*" to guide my judgment instead of my gut feelings by:
6. I will introduce the importance of realizing our personal "*why*" to my organization like this:
7. My timeline:

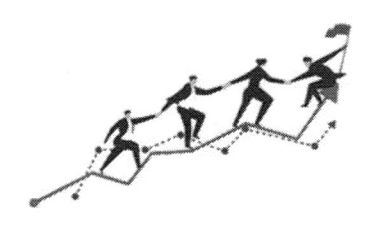

———

CHAPTER 8

RENOVATING TO REALIZE VOICE: APPRECIATING YOUR BRAND

We've Been Guilty of This

Seeing Ralph as a highly motivated leader, I couldn't help but notice how he'd placed a lot of effort into emulating the leadership style of one of his more successful colleagues. By mimicking this approach, Ralph undoubtedly believed it would somehow guarantee his success as well. We've all been guilty of this (at least I have). I've observed that many people think this way. Seeing someone else aligning the values they promote with their actions can be attractive and motivating.

Yet, the irony is we're more motivated to perform at our best when we're authentic to who we are. If you're a parent, you probably tell your children to just be themselves—as long as it's the best version of them, that doesn't wake up at 5:00 a.m. and fingerpaint the walls with peanut butter. But is this good advice for the workplace too? Of course. If authenticity is that important, why emulate someone else? This chapter will teach you how to renovate the plagiarized voice so you can realize and appreciate your own.

The Leader's Voice

Granted, the notion of a leader's voice is somewhat abstract. Your core values, vision, strengths, and behaviors, combined with how they impact your demeanor, approach, confidence, and genuineness, are what my company refers to as your leadership voice. It's who you are apart from your leadership role and your personality in performance. The combinations of thoughts and behaviors are limitless because we are all different.

Some leaders lead with their hearts and emotions, while others lead with behaviors that work against them in terms of realizing their goals. For example, some leaders will go far and wide to be right. And then there are leaders who knowingly and unknowingly design long-standing silos and "us-vs.-them" dynamics.

Some leaders inspire the imaginations of those they lead. There are coaching leaders, mentoring leaders, do-as-I-say leaders, assertive and direct leaders, trusting leaders, and distrusting leaders. Some leaders are unrelenting taskmasters. Out of this hodge-podge of behaviors emerges your leadership voice. It's your expression. It defines you. It's what others hear and respond to, positively or negatively. It's your brand. Your voice punctuates your leadership style and directly affects your team's faith in you. Oftentimes, leaders want to be like other leaders. But renovating the old to realize your voice enables you to fully step into your role with creativity, courage, and confidence and be fully present.

CHAPTER 8: Renovating To Realize Voice: Appreciating Your Brand

Why Renovate to Realize Voice

As seen earlier, Ralph felt secure in emulating the leadership style of one of his colleagues. He wasn't aware of his personal powerful leadership tools that could drive effective communication and help him articulate his vision. I'm not referring to his tone or speaking style, but the power of connecting core values, vision, strengths, and communication skills, which impacts how he shows up as a leader. He didn't realize that his *fighting-ego* was robbing his confidence in learning so much about himself and having the impact and influence he desired. No one wants to lead as a robot-like, efficient copy machine.

Let me point to a powerful illustration. Dr. Martin Luther King, Jr. was a charismatic leader who used powerful direct oratory, an engaging personality, and an unwavering commitment to positive change in the lives of millions of people. He was able to communicate peace on a deeper level. In return, he was awarded a Nobel Peace Prize.

In contrast, Mother Teresa was a very warm, gentle, and soft-spoken situational leader who generally shunned the limelight. She also had a heartfelt determination and commitment to helping people. She inspired others to join her in that effort. In return, she became known as a famous humanitarian and was also awarded a Nobel Peace Prize. Both Dr. King and Mother Teresa led in their respective professions from a place of absolute authenticity. Others followed them as a result.

Why then are we motivated to emulate someone else's voice? According to *The Oxford Handbook of Human Action*, some of our motives to act are biological, while others have personal and social origins. We are motivated to seek food, water, and sex, but our behavior is also influenced by social approval, acceptance, the need to achieve, and the motivation to take or avoid risks, to name a few.[1]

I discovered a clear example of this motivation to emulate someone else's voice when I encountered Mary at a New York City financial corporation. As the only female senior leader in our division, Mary's personal and social motives were obvious. Instead of showing up more authentic in her feminine traits—natural strengths—like being vulnerable, empathetic, collaborative, and intuitive, she succumbed to her *fighting-ego*. Mary showed up with an aggressive, authoritative, masculine leadership voice, hoping to fit in. This wasn't who she was.

One reason to remain authentic is that it's more effective because, like others, I saw through this. There was a soft, sweet, caring, yet strong person beneath all of that. Unfortunately, Mary was driven to succeed at the expense of losing all semblance of her essential self. Her unique strengths, contributions, and voice were lost and forgotten in the seemingly endless climb to get a seat at the table. Sadly, with the loss of her voice, the table was inaccessible.

Not Only Women

Male leaders have their secret motivations too. The role of provider, traditionally fallen to men pushes them to always be available, ambitious, often exhausted and not daring to show any emotion through it all. Losing their voices to their *fighting-egos* for the sake of leading like a warrior and doing whatever it takes to get the numbers, they're often frustrated with their inability to empower themselves and their teams. Never would they be seen in a softer, more authentic, and balanced way, acknowledging that their wins manifested despite their egos, not because of them.

Partnering with both male and female leaders across several different industries has shown me how organizations often weigh in by unofficially operating with a very conventional, middle-of-the-road style of leadership. Leaders want to succeed, but to avoid controversy, as their survival mechanism, they "go along with the flow," doing what others have done,

CHAPTER 8: Renovating To Realize Voice: Appreciating Your Brand

expecting to move up in the company—sounds like my experience in Chapter 1, doesn't it? All the while, the *fighting-ego* is hijacking their authentic voice. The consequential impact of this political and organizational structure is its leaders' values, visions, strengths, and talents—their voices—are reduced to a normative, predictable pattern of behavior. Organizations like these ultimately suffer too.

When you tear down the walls of emulating and mimicking, you can proactively design and build on your strengths and competencies. This will help develop the capacity for authentic leadership and a willingness to be vulnerable. Not only does this allow you the freedom to be your true self but also enables you to establish more trusting relationships and ultimately improves personal and corporate performance.

Tearing Down the Myths

Myth: Authentic leaders can say whatever comes to mind

I believe authentic leadership is often misunderstood. Merriam-Webster defines authenticity as "real or genuine; not false imitation; true to one's character." Here's Alexandra's illustrative story of how this definition becomes a reality:

> *Leaders of all types were recently at the Vistage Executive Summit in New York, and I had the privilege of attending with The Predictive Index's CEO, Mike Zani. Mike and I were able to catch the last speaker of the day. I sat in my chair, shoulders back, body bent slightly forward at attention, ankles crossed. Mike relaxed more in his seat.*
>
> *A man walked on stage, poised and in front of a large photograph, well-coiffed and better-tailored. His arms were wide as he commanded his audience. His photographs were breathtaking, but his storytelling was even better, and he grew more confident with each photograph he*

shared: Putin, Trump, and other notables—a veritable display of power in all degrees and facets. And then, there was Muhammad Ali, whose power was trapped in a body that no longer could stand toe-to-toe with its former glory. Next, a military widow, clad in her fallen husband's T-shirt, mourning that it had been washed before she could smell him one last time.

I sat there, stoic, performing the kind of composure I believed was expected of me in a room among leaders. To my right, Mike gently wiped away tears, head tilted downward, body slouched slightly forward, unconcerned with performance. At that moment, his leadership was human. It was authentic. It was impactful.
(By Alexandra LeBlanc, The Predictive Index, With Permission)

What do you see in Alexandra's experience? She recognized that a more authentic, less conventional leadership approach, as Mike demonstrated, didn't detract from his presence. With his head tilted down and his body slouched forward in his seat, Mike was unconcerned about mirroring the performance of other leaders in the room. In a vulnerable moment, not only did he push back on the trigger of his *fighting-ego*, he allowed his emotions to reveal he was human before he was a leader.

And Alexandra learned from this experience that authentic leadership is more impactful than conventional approaches. Think about this. Instead of hiding behind their emotions, authentic leaders seek to understand them. Authentic leaders are constantly seeking self-awareness. This self-awareness is developed as they become more skillful in adapting their authentic style without compromising their character or their true voice. Authenticity requires vulnerability, which most people's *fighting-ego* runs away from. Go ahead and give yourself permission to be human.

CHAPTER 8: Renovating To Realize Voice: Appreciating Your Brand

Myth: Vulnerable and transparent leaders are weak

Many believe a leader must be stoic and infallible. But it's perfectly fine to admit when you don't know something, or you tried something and failed. We want our leaders to be courageous enough to show their vulnerability.

Vulnerability is not about weakness but about showing confidence, inner strength, and transparency. Here's the secret: vulnerability feels like weakness but looks like courage to those around you. Simon Sinek, the author of *Start with Why*, clarifies what it means to be transparent in business: "Transparency doesn't mean showing everybody everything. Transparency means providing context to the decisions we make. It means keeping people in the loop."[2]

And vulnerability researcher Brené Brown describes vulnerability as "the core of all emotions and feelings; to see it as a weakness would be to conclude that feeling is failing. I define vulnerability as emotional risk, exposure, and uncertainty. It fuels our daily lives."[3]

Pete Bowen, a former AV-8B Harrier pilot and instructor in the US Marine Corps, who today is a high-performance leadership consultant, shared with me his military experience on how vulnerability can be a strength. He said, "Back in the 1990s, AV-8B Harriers were the most challenging jet to fly for a variety of reasons. We lost a lot of pilots. It became part of the culture to share the mistakes made—even stupid ones—as a way for everyone to remember, 'There but for the grace of God go I.' At pilot meetings, my commanding officer would start by sharing a mistake he made the week prior. Other pilots shared their mistakes. Transparency became the culture and helped us uncover problems. It saved lives. We didn't trust pilots who weren't transparent because it was egotistical, selfish, and put everyone at risk."

As you now can see, authenticity, vulnerability, and transparency are indeed the power strengths, not weaknesses, that enable you to have the desired and needed impact and influence. With them, there's no need to mimic another leader's voice or model another's style.

Through all the fake debris, finding your voice as a leader is the difference between becoming a mediocre executive or a dynamic, influential role model. It doesn't end with who you are but what you do with who you are. It's who you are as a person that serves you as a leader. You must be willing and able to be flexible in terms of your leadership style and methods—and so must the rest of the leaders in your organization. For example, leaders are sometimes called on to simultaneously direct multiple groups of people, and that means finding ways to effectively engage with different personality types.

FIVE PRINCIPLES OF RENOVATING TO REALIZE VOICE

Authenticity, vulnerability, and transparency are the fabrics and textures of relationships and the lens through which others experience you and your true leadership voice. An invaluable growth opportunity comes as you renovate a fake leadership voice and find ways to tap into your true voice to enhance the way you are truly perceived by others. I suggest these five principles for renovating to realize your voice.

1. *Realize your authenticity and openness*

Ann Fudge, who serves on several corporate boards, including those of General Electric, Novartis, Unilever, and Infosys, said, "Authenticity and knowing who you are is fundamental to being an effective and long-standing leader." Lance Secretan, the founder of The Secretan Center, Inc. and renowned leadership teacher, wrote, "Authenticity is the alignment of head, mouth, heart, and feet—thinking, saying, feeling, and doing the same thing—consistently. This builds trust, and followers love leaders they can trust." And Henna Inam, author of *Wired for Authenticity: Seven Practices to Inspire, Adapt, & Lead*, wrote, "Authentic leadership is the full expression of 'me' for the benefit of 'we.'"

CHAPTER 8: Renovating To Realize Voice: Appreciating Your Brand

How often do you step outside of yourself to examine if you're comfortable in your leadership skin? How often do you allow your heart to overrule your *fighting-ego*, or even what's in your head and briefcase?

Here's what you need to do:

Stand up to the *fighting-ego* trap, having the courage to explore who you are as a person. Be conscientious about your leadership responsibilities, recognizing that your title is inconsequential. You get to serve as a leader at the discretion of those whom you lead. Commit to authentically articulating a vision and giving it context through smart habits, the right goals, delivering feedback, mentoring, listening, supporting, and coaching. You will begin to realize a deeper understanding of your leadership voice.

2. *Realize your idiosyncrasies*

I have yet to know a leader who has no quirks or unconscious habits. It's what makes us who we are. We have our unique ways of serving or empowering our employees. You may be passion-oriented, vision-oriented, detail-oriented, or quiet and reserved. Martin Lanik, the author of *The Leader Habit,* wrote, "The latest brain science shows that about half of our behavior every day is automatic, based on sheer habits, like brushing our teeth, or fastening our seat belt when we get into a car."[4] These vulnerabilities can be both an asset and a liability. We can fall into automatic negative patterns, not realizing how others are impacted.

Here's what you need to do:

Strip the *fighting-ego* derailers of their power, paying close attention to your uniqueness. Look inward, be honest about your strengths and weaknesses, what qualities have worked for you in the past, and what you can improve on. You may be loud or quiet, all about productivity, or strict on being organized and punctual. Realizing your leadership voice means respecting your uniqueness, managing your extremes, and understanding your non-negotiables.

3. Realize others' perspectives

This means realizing that your leadership voice is aided by inclusion and collaboration. Everyone has a unique perspective. George S. Patton stated, "If everyone is thinking alike, then somebody isn't thinking." If we want to realize our leadership voice, we must realize that there's more than one side to a story and invite the perspectives of others. Defined in the Social Interdependence Theory of Johnson and Johnson (1989), perspective-taking communicates that one understands others' thoughts, feelings, and needs.[5] The voice of a command-and-control leader leaves little or no room for others to be heard.

Here's what you need to do:

Leadership success often depends on your ability to be tactful, develop empathy, and make an effort to appreciate other people's points of view. When you stop assuming that others share your perspective simply because you're leading and become open to their knowledge, then the walls of your *fighting-ego* will come tumbling down. The best decisions are made and easier to implement when the combined knowledge of multiple perspectives is involved.

4. Realize other people matter

Your leadership voice is stronger and more effective when you're approachable. Your voice can't be heard otherwise. Your voice can turn away or shut down an employee that approaches you with a situation, translating your voice into "you don't matter." Conversely, in a moment of transparency, inviting a conversation and giving your full attention translates your leadership voice into "you matter." This is a powerful way to manage day-to-day interruptions effectively and respectively. Chris Peterson, one of the 100 most cited psychologists in the world and one of the founding fathers of positive psychology, would open every talk and workshop by saying, "Other people matter." Peterson knew that people benefit when we let them know that they matter. And we do too.[6]

CHAPTER 8: Renovating To Realize Voice: Appreciating Your Brand

Here's what you need to do:

Show others you're consciously aware of them. Don't consider what just happened or what will happen. Allow your leadership voice to empower those you lead. Leave people better than you found them. Break through the internal walls of your *fighting-ego* to enable your unconditional style to communicate that other people matter, because they do.

5. *Realize your commitment to your vision*

Team members can easily buy into your vision when you're committed and communicate it clearly. Your voice can stay strong throughout the day-to-day craziness of business. Realistic optimism protects you by allowing you to remain confident while accepting the reality of difficult situations. This guides your leadership voice and protects you from worrying and descending into the negative leadership voice of panic, fear, and indecisiveness. People will feed off the colors of your confidence.

Here's what you need to do:

Adopt a mental tagline to keep in mind for communicating what the company is striving for, such as "vision first" or "confidence tops arrogance." It prevents the anxiety associated with a fight-or-flight or knee-jerk reaction when faced with tough situations.

Lead2Flourish Keys

1. Your leadership voice reflects your core values, vision, strengths, and behaviors, such as presence, demeanor, attentiveness, engagement, decisiveness, approach, confidence, humility, and genuineness, which impact how you present yourself as a leader.

2. Realizing your voice enables you to fully step into your role with creativity, courage, and confidence and be fully present.
3. Authenticity, vulnerability, and transparency are the life forces of relationships and the lens through which others experience you and your true leadership.

Questions for Reflection

Think back over your career and recall those times when you were inspired to act and behave by your *fighting-ego* and when you consciously followed your authentic voice.

1. Under what circumstances do I tend to emulate other successful leaders?
2. When I'm leading with my authentic voice, I feel _____
3. When I'm leading with my authentic voice, others seem to _____
4. I'm motivated to perform at my best when I _____
5. I've learned that my leadership voice makes a difference by _____

Designing a Lead2Flourish Plan – Renovating to Realize Voice

Reflecting on what you've learned in this chapter, design a plan that bonds core values, vision, and communication skills with your authentic leadership voice.

1. The counterproductive leadership behaviors to be aware of are:
2. To combat the tendency to emulate the style of other leaders, I can:
3. I make a quality decision to commit to:
4. The reasons I've made this decision are:

CHAPTER 8: Renovating To Realize Voice: Appreciating Your Brand

5. Potential *fighting-ego* hurdles:
6. I will use my authentic voice to guide my leadership style and affect my team's faith in me by:
7. I will introduce the importance of realizing voice to my organization by:
8. My timeline:

STAGE 3

REBUILDING

After renovating, it's time to rebuild. Just as the structural and mechanical plans must carry the weight of a building's designated activities, in this stage we'll rebuild the often overlooked and unrefined attributes of your core strengths, emotional resilience, and unhelpful habits to equip you to carry the weight of your day-to-day duties, performance, and pursuits.

CHAPTER 9

REBUILDING WITH SIGNATURE STRENGTHS: STRENGTH-CENTERED LEADERSHIP

Faulty or Unfaulty

Now that you've recognized the root causes of unconscious behaviors and renovated what's needed to bring together your vision, values, and voice, I want to share other attributes you can cultivate to optimize performance wellbeing. In this chapter, we refer to the first attribute as *signature strengths*. Consider this: the electrical power on one side of a building remains on all the time with no problem, but the power shorted out over time on the other side.

As an electrical engineer, how would you learn the best techniques for restoring power? Would you study the faulty wiring that shorted out over time or how the unfaulty wiring remained strong over time? I hope your answer is the latter. Yet, leaders believe they must study and try to fix weaknesses—what went wrong or what's broken. All the while, it's the strengths of the matter that keep things going.

The Science

It seems logical to seek out what went wrong in hopes of finding a solution. That's because our brains are hardwired for the negative. Researchers have argued that there is an evolutionary component to why we focus more on what's wrong than on what's right. It goes back thousands of years ago to when our ancestors were exposed to immediate environmental threats that we no longer need to worry about today—predators, for example. Being more attentive to these negative stimuli played a useful role in their survival.

Further research found that our brains respond more intensely to negative stimuli, referred to as *negativity bias*.[1] This means that your brain is wired to place greater emphasis on the negative (we saw a similar concept with Mary, Ben, Jerry, and Travis, where what went wrong in childhood triggers our behavior as an adult). Bad is stronger (more attention-getting) than good. When given one part positive and one part negative, the brain will focus on the negative. For example, people react more strongly to losing $10 than finding a $10 bill; or will have a stronger reaction to receiving criticism than praise.[2]

Leaders often believe their role is to analyze problems, brainstorm possible solutions, and then implement the best approach. As a result, you become skilled at studying what's wrong. Most consulting companies have traditionally relied on this problem-solving model. I'd like to introduce a different way to improve results that is often ignored.

CHAPTER 9: Rebuilding With Signature Strengths: Strength-Centered Leadership

Signature Strengths Explained

Signature or character strengths are the positive parts of our personality that impact how we think, feel, and behave. Our strengths provide a lens through which others can see what makes us unique. Signature strengths are the strongest or most prominent in your strengths. Ultimately, they are likely to be the strengths that matter most to you and are central to your identity.

These attributes reflect who you are at your core and are different from your other personal strengths, such as your unique skills, talents, interests, and resources. Even though different strengths predict different outcomes, accessing and expressing signature or character strengths links to important components of individual and social wellbeing. While this may be unfamiliar territory to many people, from the research and studies across cultures, we can identify and use signature strengths to consciously lead effectively.

Rebuilding Bold Leadership

No one wants to be a failure. No one wants to get it wrong. For this reason, leaders spend a lot of time fixing things, closing gaps, and solving problems. Slow down! I like how Professor Martin Seligman clarifies this: "Working hard to manage weaknesses, while sometimes necessary, will only help us prevent failure. It will not help us reach excellence." What about shifting your attention to what's already going right and working with that?

It's important to emphasize here that you may have the faulty assumption that bold leadership is about you, your leadership, and how others should get in line with you. Here's where you'd better restrain that *fighting-ego*. The reality is that strength-centered leadership turns the focus away from you to strengths that meet the needs of others. In doing this, you influence and sharpen the potential of others to become more of who they could be.

Strength-centered leadership isn't a goal to be set. It isn't something you create. It's something that's discovered and cultivated to meet the basic needs of others in the categories of trust, compassion, stability, and hope. You do this by making your strengths work for you. But how?

1. **Find out what's right with you.**

Learning to tap into the potentialities within you can be an exciting task. Your signature strengths define what you do well. This never grows old. Yes, you have the chance to do what you do best every day! The Gallup Organization asked this question of 198,000 employees working in 7,939 business units within 36 companies: "At work, do you have the opportunity to do what you do best every day?" It was more predictive of low employee turnover, high employee engagement, and high employee success rate than other questions, such as, "Are you satisfied with your pay?"[3]

Here's what you need to do:

Your greatest room for growth is in the areas of your greatest strength. Only then can you appreciate and leverage the strengths of others. Here's where to start.

- Observe when you're at your best, in your zone, flowing in what you do, and energized by it. Then ask your colleagues and family to observe you in the same way. Their recurring responses are your strengths.

- Complete the Virtues in Action (VIA®) Inventory of Strengths Survey at www.viacharacter.org. The VIA conceptualizes strengths as morally valued components of character that contribute to a fulfilling life (Peterson & Seligman, 2004). Upon completion, you will get your free results immediately and can print them out. You'll have the option to purchase a more detailed report for $40. Pay attention to the rank order of your strengths. Next, look at your five highest strengths and ask yourself of each, "Is it a *signature* strength?"

- Complete the CliftonStrengths online assessment at gallup.com and receive your strengths package for $10. The CliftonStrengths

CHAPTER 9: Rebuilding With Signature Strengths: Strength-Centered Leadership

measures the intensity of your talents in each of its thirty-four themes that represent what people do best. It views strengths as personal competencies that generate optimal performance. Pay attention to your top five strengths.

- You can also purchase the book *StrengthsFinder* 2.0 (Rath) or *Strengths Based Leadership: Great Leaders, Teams and Why People Follow* (Rath and Conchie). An access code in the back of the book will allow you to take the online assessment and receive your complete strengths report at no additional cost.

2. **Find out what brings life to you and life to others.**

Are you a leader who kills motivation and potential by telling your employees, "Don't approach me with a problem unless you can offer a solution." Reframe your language to enhance the positive and energize both you and the receiver. Let them know you are that leader who understands what it means to serve others. In a previous chapter, I shared an incident where a former boss called me to his office and approached me in an accusatory manner. If my boss had adopted a strength-centered approach, he would not have overreacted but responded in a way that enlivened both of us and the situation. For example, discussing the matter with me privately and thoroughly would have built the trust I needed.

Here's what you need to do:

First, deepen your understanding of how your strengths influence others. Then focus on how your strengths meet the needs of others. It's important here that you focus on solutions, not the problems. Show your followers it's psychologically safe to come to you even with undesirable news. Without blaming, ask strength-centered questions such as, "Do you understand how we got here? What do you see as a short-term and long-term solution? What have we already done so that we can replicate this time? What can we do to prevent this from recurring?"

3. **Discuss outcomes you wish to see instead of talking about what's wrong.**

We live in a world that our questions create. When leaders change their questions, everything can change.

Here's what you need to do:

Instead of questioning the negative or what's going wrong, apply the same attention to studying and furthering what's going right. You take this approach when studying the competition, don't you? The *fighting-ego* will push back and resist this approach because it's accustomed to improving results by looking at problems. The research of Columbia University psychology and business professor E. Tory Higgins found that when people focus on what they most desire and remind themselves of their ideals and aspirations, they're more energized to make changes and take action. Evaluating exceptional results optimizes you to make changes and act rather than evaluating problems and areas of caution.[4]

THREE PRINCIPLES OF REBUILDING WITH SIGNATURE STRENGTHS

The dual purpose of becoming aware of your signature strengths is that you become more of who you are to unlock your potential while aligning your strengths to meet the needs of others and influence them to become more of who they could be. Rebuild with signature strengths with these three principles in mind.

1. Audit yourself

Deepen your understanding of who you are while reviewing your strengths profile. Science shows that people who find new ways to use their strengths throughout their day are happier and less depressed.[5]

CHAPTER 9: Rebuilding With Signature Strengths: Strength-Centered Leadership

Here's what you need to do:

Focus on amplifying the good in yourself, your life, and those around you. Recognize the times when you use your strengths. Focus on using them in new ways. Mindfully use your strengths, including them in all your behaviors, actions, activities, and interactions. Be mindful of the jolt of your *fighting-ego* to react. Respond instead with your strengths.

2. *Enliven yourself*

Appreciate the wonderful qualities you bring to the world. This helps you with confidence and self-assurance, which makes you less likely to compare yourself to others.

Here's what you need to do:

Use your best qualities in novel ways. This helps you to discover different parts of yourself and what you're capable of doing. Intentionally notice how you use your strengths to contribute to those around you positively.

3. *Influence and enliven others*

This, in my view, is a strength in itself. Influencing and enlivening others mean reaching deeper with your strengths to meet their needs.

Here's what you need to do:

When others share a good idea, recognize their perspective and creativity. Be grateful for their input and comment on their innovation. Labeling the signature strength gives the person new insight into their activities, and expressing appreciation allows the person to feel that their strengths matter.[6] Allow yourself to rely on others more by learning where their greatest potential lies and how partnering with them increases the influence and engagement in each of you.

What Follows After Knowing Your Strengths?

Being a resourceful leader requires a deep understanding of your strengths. Seligman and Petersen suggested that every person possesses three to seven out of twenty-four signature strengths, which represent the core of the person's identity. Being aware of your strengths is one thing. Knowing how to use your strengths is what follows.

Having a coach is one of the most time-effective ways of developing leadership. A 2014 study found that when thirty-seven executives and managers received workplace coaching over three months, their leadership skills improved significantly.[7] Strength-centered coaching offers a practical approach to finding your strengths and developing existing and future leaders. Once you understand how to use your strengths, you are ready to introduce this concept to your team and employees.

Lead2Flourish Keys

1. Many leaders believe their role is to analyze problems, brainstorm possible solutions, and then implement the best approach. As a result, you become skilled at studying what's wrong. A more effective approach is studying what's right.
2. Your signature strength defines what you do well. Your greatest room for growth is in the areas of your greatest strength.
3. Strength-centered leadership helps to meet the basic needs of followers in the categories of trust, compassion, stability, and hope.
4. Discuss outcomes you wish to see instead of talking about what's wrong.
5. Strength-centered coaching offers a practical approach to finding your strengths and developing existing and future leaders.

CHAPTER 9: Rebuilding With Signature Strengths: Strength-Centered Leadership

Questions for Reflection

1. Name a strength-centered approach you can use instead of "analyzing the problem."
2. Explain how you will "build on what's right" instead of "fixing what's wrong."
3. Why is it important to focus on the solution and not the problem?
4. Is there an opportunity to do what you do best every day?
5. What are your intrinsic motivators for rebuilding with strength-centered leadership?

Designing a Lead2Flourish Plan – Rebuilding With Signature Strengths

Reflecting on what you learned in this chapter, design a plan from who you are at your core to meet the needs of others.

1. I tend to focus on what went wrong when I:
2. I've decided to commit to:
3. The reasons I've made this decision are:
4. Potential fighting-ego hurdles:
5. Here's my plan to rebuild with signature strengths and focus them on helping others:
6. Here's how I plan to introduce strength-centered leadership to my organization:
7. My timeline:

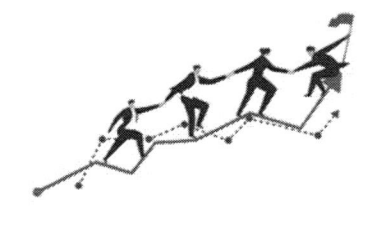

CHAPTER 10

REBUILDING WITH EMOTIONAL RESILIENCE: ENERGIZED LEADERSHIP

Keeping the Sails Steady

Sandra had served only four months of a three-year contract that would allow her to commission as an officer in the United States Army. Less than one percent of Americans achieve this task. Sandra was striving to be included in that one percent. But Sandra had a secret. Pushing against her *fighting-ego* as her heart beat fast and hands sweated, she drove to her Master Sergeant's office to inform him of her secret—she was pregnant.

Sandra told her Master Sergeant she'd need to take off the fall semester but planned to return the following semester after her child was born.

Expecting his usual upbeat, encouraging response, instead, his words stung hard. "Sandra, be honest; you're not coming back. Statistics show that most women who get pregnant while in this program do not return to finish. I think it would be easier for you to drop out and return home." But Sandra was incredibly determined. After the birth of her son, she returned to complete the program and took her oath of office, confirming her commission as a leader in the United States Army.

Angie was an urban planner who'd recently transferred from the private sector of local government to work in its public sector. Her new colleagues had worked there for decades. Although she was bright, intelligent, and hardworking, with new ideas and approaches, her seasoned colleagues openly and unashamedly rejected her input. Angie tolerated the brash outbursts and rejection for over eighteen months. As a team player, she dared not go outside of her team circle to handle any disputes. She was targeted for bullying but didn't allow her *fighting-ego* to overshadow her love for her work.

Angie purposefully learned to detach her emotions from the conflicts. When Angie made a career change, she used the bullying experiences as a catalyst to become a passionate and effective leader. In Angie's words, "Resilient leaders can take a hit to the chin and stand strong while delivering a round-nose punch."

Sandra and Angie rose with the strength to power through the storm and kept their sails steady. How? By what *Psychology Today's* chief editor, Hara Estroff Marano, refers to as "an art of living that is entwined with self-belief, self-compassion, and enhanced cognition, empowering themselves to perceive these adversities as temporary, evolving through the pain and sufferings and not letting it affect their internal motivation to uncover one of the most important behaviors of a leader—emotional resilience."

CHAPTER 10: Rebuilding With Emotional Resilience: Energized Leadership

Responding to Your Pain

Your responsibilities as a leader include sustaining wellbeing and high performance both for yourself and your people. We've recognized how the *fighting-ego* cycle can add pressure and bring on stressful and unpredictable disruptions. You can react in one of three ways—explode emotionally, implode helplessly, or respond purposely by using your core strengths to power through and keep the sail steady. Moreover, humans are capable of and creative at resolving issues and can become stronger and more flexible in stressful times. Psychologists call this *emotional resilience*, and it's a key factor in sailing through pressure and stress and performing at your highest level.

You've heard about resilience. You might know about resilience. But did you know that without it, you and your organization will not consistently reach higher goals or lead from a place of courage, wisdom, and strength? The events of 2020 through 2022 have shown that our lives may also be impacted by great trauma. The choice here is whether you should react on a whim, wallow in an adverse situation, or respond with confidence while keeping your sails steady. In this chapter, we are undoing unconscious behaviors and rebuilding with emotional resilience—what I call *bouncing forward*, and not bouncing back, from adverse experiences.

Emotional resilience is the ability to calm your frantic mind after encountering an undesirable experience. It's an inner force, intrinsic motivation by which you can hold yourself through all of life's setbacks.

Understanding and neutralizing counterproductive unconscious behaviors is an important step toward becoming a flourishing leader. Doing so without also understanding and accounting for emotional resilience, however, won't get you all the way there. Emotional resilience is a critical component of flourishing leadership.

Opening to Emotional Resilience

According to the research of Karen Reivich, PhD, and Andrew Shatte, Ph.D., what makes one person resilient and another not is often *determined during childhood*. How we analyze events depends on thinking styles that we have learned over our lifetime that operate reflexively, in knee-jerk fashion, when things don't go our way. Non-resilient thinking styles can lead us to cling to inaccurate beliefs about the world and to inappropriate problem-solving strategies that burn through emotional energy and valuable resilience resources.[1]

If you were to be fired from your job, your emotions would try to take over, but you'd still start looking for another job, wouldn't you? Even if you were offered a less desirable position, you'd override your *fighting-ego* and take the job because you need the money as soon as possible. Emotional resilience would kick in as a reflex when facing a predicament such as this.

Let's say, in a less threatening, day-to-day situation, your colleague got the promotion that was promised to you, you got into a heated argument with your spouse, or your flat tire caused you to be late for an important meeting. What would you choose to do in these scenarios? Collect yourself to exercise emotional resilience, or without thinking, react with rage, allowing your *fighting-ego* to take control?

And wait just a minute before you answer that question. I want you to beware that in addition to the common experiences that require resilience to survive, we often need to be resilient even in the face of positive changes. Yes, that's right! Now imagine that your company has just initiated a re-organization. You already know you'll have a better position there, but you'll also have a new manager, most of your team members will be new, and your responsibilities are likely to change substantially. This is a positive change, isn't it? As university psychologists, Carolyn Youssef and Fred Luthans have discovered, having increased responsibilities, forward progress, and significant positive events can all result in the need for adaptation and recovery. The response to positive change also highlights the need for emotional resilience.[2]

There's good news. Resilience is not a gene that people either have or do not have. It involves behaviors, thoughts, and actions that can be learned and developed by anyone.[3] Though one person may have a natural tendency toward resilience, it ultimately comes down to choice. And choices are voluntary, although they may not always feel like it in the heat of the moment. The greater you can understand your emotions, the greater you can change them. When you know your emotions, you gain greater resilience in your life.

Rebuilding With Emotional Resilience

> *"Resilience is a muscle. Flex it enough, and it will take less effort to get over the emotional punches each time."* —Alecia Moore

Rebuilding with emotional resilience is a matter of being aware of your inner potential. What differentiates an emotionally resilient and an emotionally fragile leader is the way the former chooses to respond. Emotional resilience doesn't mean that stress won't affect you or losses won't depress you. It only implies that you still have the vision to stand up and keep moving ahead. With clarification, the late, renowned psychologist Chris Petersen referred to resilience as the ability to "struggle well." Learning to struggle well is not an invitation to tolerate fallbacks and adversities at work. But rather, it's a gateway to flourishing. Here's why.

Resilience is an important behavior in the context of work. Every leader will, at some point, receive negative feedback, or experience a failure or change at work. This fact of life highlights the role of a leader's emotional resilience. By recognizing where we have failed or come up short, we can identify the most constructive ways to move forward with strength and the enthusiasm to get it right the next time. Psychologist and professor Adam

Grant put it this way: "Resilience is not a race to bounce back from hardship. It's a commitment to keep going in the face of hardship." With emotional resilience, we can work through the effects of pressure, anxiety, and negative emotions and not only bounce forward but flourish.

Emotional resilience helps us to develop our skills and interact effectively with others. It impacts our motivation, cognitive functioning, and wellbeing. A serious lack of emotional resilience can lead to helplessness and seeing ourselves as a victim of circumstance. For example, a fear of public speaking may cause us to remain silent even when we know we have something to contribute to a discussion. Another example is if we become defensive when receiving negative feedback, we can forgo the opportunity to learn and develop our skills. Sounds like Jackie's story in Chapter 5, doesn't it? An important aspect of rebuilding with emotional resilience is its link with other life domains. This means building resilience at work would also make you resilient in your relationships and vice versa.

SIX PRINCIPLES OF REBUILDING WITH EMOTIONAL RESILIENCE

Understand that you are not at the mercy of your emotions. You have more control over your emotions than you may believe. Your brain is wired so that if you change what it uses to create emotion, then it can adapt to changes that never existed in your life before. Keep the following principles in mind as you rebuild with emotional resilience to bounce forward, not bounce back.

1. *Emotional resilience is your responsibility*

Displacing how you feel by looking for others to take emotional responsibility is not uncommon. We must take responsibility for ourselves. Taking responsibility for ourselves includes accepting responsibility for our thoughts, our feelings, our emotions, our actions, and their consequences.

CHAPTER 10: Rebuilding With Emotional Resilience: Energized Leadership

Because emotions are contagious, being irresponsible with an emotional outburst can trigger a corresponding or complementary emotion in others.

Here's what you need to do:

Contain the emotions by observing your reactions. Containing does not mean suppressing or denying your emotions. Start with journaling a detailed description of yourself as a whole person: physically, mentally, emotionally, spiritually, and relationally. When you contain the emotions, you experience the emotion, just as Sandra and Angie did, but the emotion doesn't trigger you to react or do the talking. The part of your mind that's in charge takes over. That's emotional responsibility in action. But be warned, it won't be easy. You will often find yourself faced with contradictions, given that your *fighting-ego* will want to protect itself.

2. Broken pieces drive growth

As you rebuild with emotional resilience, you not only adapt to stress and disappointments, but you also grow the insight to avoid reacting and engaging behaviors that might lead you to face future situations.

Here's what you need to do:

Maintain awareness of your emotions and a keen determination to learn from any slip-ups. This awareness is what helps you to grow and connect with your psychological and physiological needs—knowing what you need, what you don't need, and when it's time to reach out for some extra help. Also, you'll cultivate awareness of the subtle cues your body and mood are sending.

3. Self-care is healthcare

Self-care habits will support you when you need strength and energy. Habits to improve your physical strength, energy, health, and vitality give you the momentum to rebuild emotional resilience to weather the storm of emotional setbacks.

LEAD2FLOURISH

Here's what you need to do:

Establish self-care habits. Engage in physical activity to relieve stress. The American College of Sports Medicine (ACSM) recommends that American adults exercise for at least thirty minutes most days to improve their health and quality of life.[4] You may want to participate in physical activities that are age-appropriate, enjoyable, and offer variety. Engaging your physical strength can allow you to feel stronger emotionally to rebuild your resilience.

4. *Relational and spiritual focus builds emotional resilience*

Strong interpersonal relationships, group conformity, likeability, communication, cooperation, and spiritual energy strengthen your ability to rebuild with emotional resilience.

Here's what you need to do:

Philosopher and civil rights leader Howard Thurman said, "Don't ask what the world needs. Ask what makes you come alive and go do it. Because what the world needs is people who have come alive." Emotionally resilient leaders are in touch with what's important to them. Identify and participate in activities that make you come alive and feel happy and fulfilled. With strong interpersonal relationships, you are not alone and can use the help that is available to you. Recognize when you need help from family, friends, or anyone willing to support you. Also, identify and live up to what you value—practice what you preach.

5. *Peace is something to hold on to*

Building emotional resilience in a professional setting may seem difficult, especially when something unrelated to work itself is affecting your performance, for example, a conflict with colleagues, a loved one's sickness or death, bullying, or personal stress. You want to lash out, but rebuilding with emotional resilience involves holding on to your peace.

CHAPTER 10: Rebuilding With Emotional Resilience: Energized Leadership

Here's what you need to do:

Outsmart pressure and anxiety. Discipline your coping mechanisms. Build your resilience power. In his book, *Emotional Resilience: How to Safeguard Your Mental Health*, Cognitive Behavior expert Dr. Harry Barry says that the reason some people are better at managing stress than others is their resilience power. Exposure to toxic stress (burnout) arouses intense emotions, and our coping mechanisms are immediately deployed to manage the situation.[5] You can begin outsmarting stress and rebuilding with emotional resilience as you:

- are aware of thoughts, emotions, and inner potential
- think before reacting
- acclimatize patience and understanding
- engage acceptance and forgiveness
- focus on finding solutions
- express emotions in a socially acceptable way
- avoid bottling up negative emotions
- create and sustain long-term relationships
- aren't ashamed to ask for help when it's needed the most
- sort out conflicts through discussions

6. *Distractions are for mastering*

It takes a strong will to master distractions. It means being in the presence of the moment without judgment or avoidance. This takes practice, but it's one of the purest ways of emotional resilience building.

Here's what you need to do:

Sit in silence. You may decide to engage in quiet prayer. Close your eyes. Experience living in the now. Breathe deeply, allowing your body to relax, and your mind and emotions will follow. Deep breathing is one of the fastest ways you can get your nervous system to calm down and snap out of *the fighting-ego* reaction. Remember that by taking breaks between activities or meetings to quiet and separate yourself from what you have experienced, you can neutralize any stressful emotions.

Lead2Flourish Keys

1. Emotional resilience is a key factor in sailing through stress and performing at your highest level.
2. With a resilient attitude, you don't have to feel victimized by disruptive experiences or events in your career.
3. Emotional resilience comes when you discover what works well in you.
4. Resilience after a fallback or adverse experience is in how you respond, saying no when your fighting-ego cycle would rather react.
5. You can nurture healthy self-esteem, a positive self-concept, and strong self-confidence by reassessing who you are and your principles for living.

Questions for Reflection

1. Normally, my first thoughts when I face a difficult situation are:
   (Example: I shouldn't react to this in the heat of the moment, or it's better if I pause and purposely decide how to speak in this situation)
2. It's distressing when I feel:
   (Example: suspicious, apprehensive, see difficulties as a means to no end)
3. The underlying belief I need to question is:
   (Example: Success is mostly about how others see me)
4. I blame myself when:
   I blame others when:
   I always ask for help because:
   I never ask for help because:

CHAPTER 10: Rebuilding With Emotional Resilience: Energized Leadership

Designing a Lead2Flourish Plan – Rebuilding With Emotional Resilience

Reflecting on what you learned in this chapter, design a plan to hold yourself through all the downsides of life when encountering a negative experience and rebuild with emotional resilience.

1. Adapting to disappointments and bouncing forward will:
2. I've decided to commit to:
3. The reasons I've made this decision are:
4. Potential *fighting-ego* hurdles:
5. Here's my plan to rebuild with emotional resilience and keep the sail steady:
6. I will introduce energized leadership to my organization by:
7. My timeline:

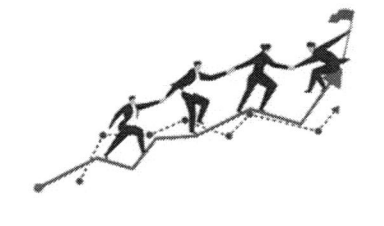

CHAPTER 11

REBUILDING WITH SMART HABITS: EFFICIENT LEADERSHIP

Vehicle of a Plan

Oftentimes, we leaders set personal performance goals for pushing the needle on our potential and productivity. But we succeed by reaching our goals. Renowned artist Pablo Picasso told us, "Our goals can only be reached through a vehicle of a plan, in which we must fervently believe, and upon which we must vigorously act. There's no other route to success." Sometimes I think we focus on the wrong vehicle. Could Picasso's *vehicle of a plan* be to vigorously act on rebuilding with smart habits? In this chapter, I'll show you why I believe this to be true.

Many of our daily behaviors are composed of little habits. These behaviors are formed unconsciously and acted out automatically. Without giving it much thought, if any at all, we repeat these routines much the same way each time. Stop reading for a moment to think about your daily routines: how you make your bed, comb your hair, or put your keys in the same pocket after you lock the door. You've repeated the same actions over and over, in similar circumstances, until it's ingrained in your brain circuitry. They're effortless habits that free your thought processes to work on more important things. Our brains are smart this way, which helps us to be more efficient.

Build Smart Habits. Achieve SMART Goals

To achieve our workplace goals, George Doran wrote in the 1981 AMA Review, "When it comes to writing effective objectives, corporate officers, managers, and supervisors just have to think of the acronym SMART." The basic acronym SMART refers to *Specific, Measurable, Attainable, Realistic, and Timely*. However, I believe strategic goals are more complex and require more than just checking off a box that fits into the SMART concept.

Consider this: If you ignored your goal of increasing revenue by 50% this month, but to reach that goal, you focused instead on your team's daily performance strategy, would you still get results? I believe you would. Then directly focusing on increasing revenue isn't necessary.

Of course, the goal of any business is to reduce waste and increase profits, but it would be ridiculous to spend every day, headstrong, only focusing on achieving the right numbers. You'd be better off identifying the "revenue triggers" and creating a series of actions for how you'll accomplish them. However, if increasing revenue is the goal or plan, then the vehicle is not the goal itself. The *vehicle of the plan* then is the actions or *habits* (performance) to achieve the goal or plan.

For most leaders I meet, building smart habits is a complicated, rarely achieved plan. Yet when studying habit creation, it's nothing short of the best use of our energy, intellect, and time. Habits aren't hard to create or change if you use science.

CHAPTER 11: Rebuilding With Smart Habits: Efficient Leadership

Habit Research

Researchers tell us that more than 40% of the actions we take are governed by habit, not actual decisions (as most leaders have determined). Habits are the way the mind naturally works to code your behavior.[1] This corresponds to what William James said: "Our virtues are habits as much as our vices ... our nervous systems have grown to the way in which they have been exercised, just as a sheet of paper or a coat, once creased or folded, tends to fall forever afterward into the same identical folds."

According to a 2009 study, it takes our brain less time to adopt smaller behaviors as habits than larger ones (like goals), suggesting that the brain more readily accepts and parses easier behaviors.[3] In many ways, habits are not only the framework of every person's life, but they define who we are and create the most efficient vehicle for achieving goals.

Transferring This Thinking to the Workplace

A lot of stress and frustration can occur from managing a team and pushing to meet goals. Kim, a client whom you met earlier in Chapter 7, was a brilliant systems analyst. One concern she had was not having enough time to get things done. As a wife, mother, and team leader, she was afraid of missing her targets, which caused longer working hours and less time with her family. Her innermost goal was to become time efficient while maintaining optimum performance and spending quality time with her family. I suggested that she take her focus off herself and her day-to-day duties (goal) and instead place emphasis on mini strategic actions (vehicle) for getting them done.

To establish these smart habits, we created a calendar with varying time slots to prompt her on what to focus on for a given period. She journaled, designating periods and procedures for carrying out her tasks. She wasn't allowed to carry over any activities to another time slot. As suspected, supported by the results of others, it worked well for Kim because the habit of writing down her daily intentions greatly increased her chances of following through. Her smart habits became embedded into her brain, and as a result, she automatically became efficient with her time, which kept her performance and family time intact.

In Chapter 1, I shared the incident where an executive put me on the spot with a client because he thought I'd neglected to follow up on something. After that episode, I set a performance goal to never be suspected of neglecting my responsibilities or being embarrassed in that way again. I started building smart habits of writing "notes to file" that documented everything I did within my assigned portfolio. I also made copies of all notes and correspondence to my clients and locked them in a "file to self" in my office.

These habits created additional steps, yet they became an effortless norm and were the smartest system I've ever built while working in the corporate landscape. Soon thereafter, other leaders were doing the same thing. As I think about it, not only was this an excellent practice that protected my reputation, but it was simply common sense. In my absence, others could pick up a file and know immediately what was going on and move forward from where I'd left off and never miss a beat.

What I Know Now

I learned from this experience that, unlike motivation alone, smart habits can auto-correct chore-like tasks into natural, automatic behaviors. While having the desire and motivation are important for making a change or, in my case, protecting my reputation, they're not enough when it comes to dealing with the temptation to forgo the effort. As Professor BJ Fogg, author of *Tiny Habits: The Small Changes That Change Everything*, explains, "When it comes to changing our behaviors, the problem is that motivation and willpower are shapeshifters by nature, which makes them unreliable." On the other hand, when smart habits become automatic, motivation and willpower are built into the process.

It's safe to say then that goals are good for planning your progress, and habits are good for making progress. One thing to realize is that attempting to reach a goal above your ability in the short term requires you to challenge your *fighting-ego* in how you currently do things. As William James once said, "Every good that is worth possessing must be paid for in strokes of daily effort." Having to make conscious decisions about everything you do all day would be strenuous for your brain. Hence, it searches for ways to be efficient by remembering actions and behaviors that are repeated consistently. Your brain stores these actions and behaviors as habits so you can follow the routine without having to think about it beforehand.

FOUR PRINCIPLES OF REBUILDING WITH SMART HABITS

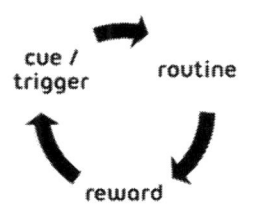

MIT researchers discovered a simple neurological loop at the core of every habit, a loop that consists of three parts: a cue, a routine, and a reward; this is known as the habit loop.[4]

Keep the following foundational principles in mind as you begin to rebuild with smart habits to achieve your goals.

1. *Psychological cues will guide your behavior*

To carry out a specific action regularly, you need a reliable reminder, a cue. Cues are the physical or mental triggers that tell your brain to follow a learned routine or habit.

Here's what you need to do:

Psychologist Robert Cialdini offers one simple way of thinking about these triggers: to use "if, then, or when" statements as a strategy for reprogramming your brain to achieve your goals.[5] For example, taking my personal story, *IF* I diligently document my performance and activities, THEN I'll have proof when someone falsely accuses me, which could potentially garner more respect. Begin by identifying a specific cue that you can use to prompt that action and reprogram your mind with if/then statements.

2. Routines are habits

Routines are the steps or the actual habits you perform, which can take the form of a thought or an action. Remember, your habits also depend on your ability. Habits can be created only if you can do them.

Here's what you need to know:

Because the cue is the first indication that you're close to a reward, it naturally leads to a desire. Desires are the motivational force behind every habit. Without some level of motivation—without desiring a change—you have no reason to act. What you desire is not the habit itself but the change it delivers (increased bottom line and possible promotion). You may decide to dedicate two or three hours of your morning to work on the goal until it's accomplished. You'll consistently continue with this routine, the habit(s), because you know there's a reward waiting for you.

3. Rewards are the benefits

Finally, the routine delivers a reward. Rewards are the benefits you receive for following those routine steps.

Here's what you need to do:

Seek the rewards, not the goal. Rewards satisfy your desires. For example, achieving the goal may bring you a promotion, more respect, or an increased salary. Rewards teach you which habits are worth remembering in the future. For example, every time you check off a task on your to-do list, your brain secretes the hormone dopamine, which corresponds with pleasure, learning, and motivation. This is what makes you feel good about yourself when you do something you intend to do. This itself is a reward.

4. *The vehicle of the plan*

Now that you know your vehicle—the habit loop—the reward that drives your behavior, the cue that triggers it, and the routine itself, you can confidently write your plan or goal.

Here's what you need to do:

Write your plan for carrying out your routine. For example, "Every day from 9:30 a.m. to 11:30 a.m., I will work on my goal." You can begin shifting the behavior from fearing time constraints, pressure, and poor performance to confidence and excitement. You can also change to a better routine by planning for the cue and choosing a behavior that delivers the reward you desire. If you abide by your plan, eventually, it becomes automatic and occurs almost without having to think about it. Then it becomes a smart habit. When you have a setback, use your emotional resilience. Change won't happen overnight. According to Charles Duhigg, "Once you understand how a habit operates, once you diagnose the cue, the routine, and the reward, you gain power over it."

Lead2Flourish Keys

1. Habits (vehicles) achieve the goal (plan).
2. Researchers tell us that more than 40% of the actions we take are governed by habit, not actual decisions. They're the way your mind naturally works to code your behavior.
3. Smart habits can auto-correct chore-like tasks into natural, automatic behaviors.
4. A simple neurological loop is at the core of every habit: a cue, a routine, and a reward known as the habit loop.
5. If you abide by your plan, eventually, it becomes automatic and occurs almost without you having to think about it. It becomes a smart habit.

Questions for Reflection

1. Think about a time when your actions were based on quick decisions rather than smart habits. What behaviors surfaced? What qualities or helpful behaviors would you have liked to develop?
2. Think of a time when you focused headstrong on a goal to reach a certain status that proved counterproductive. How different would it have been had you relied on a series of actions instead?
3. The next time you become stressed by having to reach a goal and perform well, how will you address it?

Designing a Lead2Flourish Plan: Rebuilding With Smart Habits

1. The areas where I need to build more awareness are:
2. I've decided to commit to:
3. The reasons I've made this decision are:
4. Potential *fighting-ego* hurdles:
5. My rebuilding plan to develop self-discipline is:
6. How will I introduce rebuilding with smart habits to my organization?
7. My timeline:

STAGE 4

RECHARGING

In this stage, we'll inspect your punch list as a safeguard to keep everything performing smoothly. We'll anchor and strengthen supportive behaviors using intentional self-management practices that recharge wellbeing and performance. We'll help with getting the needed alignment and efficiency to flourish at work and in life.

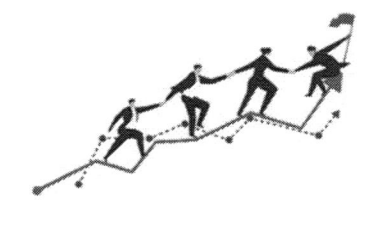

CHAPTER 12

RECHARGING THE BUSINESS OF WELLBEING: CONSCIOUS LEADERSHIP

A Positive Posture

Performance is about wellbeing. Optimizing wellbeing is about behavior. As we're increasingly successful in our behaviors, our wellbeing takes on a more positive posture. Equally, as we're increasingly successful in our wellbeing, our business takes on a more positive posture too. The more I studied behavior, wellbeing, and performance, the more clearly I was able to see the link between them. High levels of executive wellbeing create a valuable business resource. Living your life well results, in turn, in doing better business. These are not mutually exclusive. As we're positively conditioned in our behaviors, wellbeing, and performance, our business improves accordingly. This is why the business of wellbeing must be central to any business strategy.

In this chapter, I'll guide you through conscious behaviors for recharging your business of wellbeing using what I call sustainable vitality behaviors. Psychologists tell us vitality is considered an aspect of wellbeing that includes being vital, energetic, fully functioning, and psychologically well.[1]

Let's consider these descriptions of vitality behaviors: approaching life with excitement and energy, living life as an adventure, feeling alive and activated, and not doing things halfway or halfheartedly. To live this way, to perform at our highest self and inspire others to follow, we must be energetic and psychologically well. Understand that I'm referring to more than just physical activity, as there are many different ways to build vitality into your life. Here's a quick snapshot of what that looks like:

- Doing something because you want to do it, not because you feel you have to.
- Engaging in positive self-talk: "I'm the best person for closing this deal."
- Writing down the good things about your day and how you choose to live: "I'm flourishing therefore my business is flourishing."
- Going out of your way to becoming more involved in an organization to which you already belong.
- Discovering what you love to do and then building time for it in your schedule.
- Taking long nature walks, getting a good night's sleep, and eating a good breakfast to give yourself more energy during the day.

When you use strategies to create sustainable vitality behavior in building constructive thoughts, intrinsically motivated situations, and successful

CHAPTER 12: Recharging The Business Of Wellbeing: Conscious Leadership

executions, something important happens. You become an inspiration to others in the way you're able to pursue and achieve your goals.

Discovering Performance Wellbeing

At our core, we want to be well and achieve peak performance. One of the best definitions for performance I've heard is a summary term used to include the *desired behaviors and the valuable outcomes produced by those behaviors*. Another way to summarize performance is doing the necessary or required things in a way that positively contributes to personal and business goals.

I've learned that leaders can't experience high levels of work-related wellbeing without also experiencing high levels of intellectual engagement and flow with their work.

Mihaly Csíkszentmihályi found that the more time we spend doing activities in which we experience flow, the greater wellbeing we will experience.[2] Wellbeing gives us the resources to navigate the highs and lows often experienced in our work and lives, feeling in harmony—enabling us to flourish. Business is affected by our wellbeing. Wellbeing is affected by our behaviors and varies from person to person because each of us has a different combination of psychological, emotional, social, and physical resources upon which we draw.

From these descriptions, I've determined that *performance wellbeing* is a state we experience when we tap into desired behaviors that enable us to *be well, do well, and flourish* in business and life.

Watch Out for Those Subtle Behaviors

As leaders, we wear many hats. It seems there's something or someone constantly vying for our attention. Because of our time constraints, subtle behavior patterns may seem innocent and insignificant but can hijack our efforts to *be well, do well, and flourish*. We generally brush them aside because our *fighting-egos* have convinced us this is who we are and how we're wired.

But the truth is these subtle behaviors have an adverse effect and often become the norm, not the exception. Can you identify with any of these subtle behaviors?

1. *You're laboring in the service of leading*—compelled to stay busy because you like being busy. Are you finding it harder to provide the same quality of work or creative thinking when you're running around putting out fires and drowning in busyness? Driven by this behavioral pattern eventually robs your performance, productivity, happiness, burnout protection, and business goals.[3]

2. *You're more concerned with superficial things than what truly matters.* Do you keep putting things off for another day and forget your pressing needs or important goals? This unhelpful behavior can catch up with you when negative circumstances arise out of unfinished situations.

3. *You're oblivious to all the little things around you.* Is your mind all over the place, spending a lot of time planning and worrying about the future and reminiscing about the past? Doing so causes you to miss out on inspiration to perform and fails to develop your curiosities.

4. *You're addicted to your smartphone.* Do you feel left out or think you're missing out on important news or information if you don't check your phone regularly? Like the use of drugs and alcohol, this can trigger the release of the brain chemical dopamine and alter your mood. Overuse of smartphones and the internet can impact your wellbeing, taking a toll on your mental and physical health.

5. *You bite your fingernails.* Do you repetitively bite your nails while in deep thought and find it hard to control or stop? Nail biting, also known as onychophagia, is a body-focused repetitive behavior (BFRB).[4] This behavior, when uncontrolled, can cause psychological distress such as decreased self-esteem or increased anxiety.

CHAPTER 12: Recharging The Business Of Wellbeing: Conscious Leadership

6. *You subscribe to self-handicapping behaviors.* Do you frequently make excuses for having a poor attitude, a poor work performance, the fear of failure or success, or discomfort with new challenges, tasks, and duties? Leaders who subscribe to self-handicapping can develop thinking patterns that have negative consequences for their performance, wellbeing, and success.

7. *You forget to eat and hydrate your body.* Are you prone to skipping meals, not feeling hungry, and often realizing it's late at night and you haven't eaten or drunk anything in twenty-four hours? Food is the fuel that affects your energy levels, vitality, how you perform, and your long-term wellbeing.

8. *You find it difficult to get a restful night's sleep.* How many nights do you spend tossing and turning because anxious thoughts have hijacked your mind? Restful sleep is the lynchpin that helps us to sustain vitality behavior and maintain peak performance. Not having restful sleep or having poor sleeping habits has a strong effect on your overall energy and business results.

Most of these would apply to anyone. Which of these vitality-draining behaviors could be true for you? And what other subtle behaviors that aren't on this list could be true for you? Think right now about what needs are being met by subtle behaviors like these and how you can successfully replace these behaviors to meet those needs.

Research suggests most things that hurt physical health or mood also hurt vitality. For example, smoking, poor diet, inactivity, and a stressful environment are all negatively associated with vitality, and yet our vitality behavior safety is routinely neglected. Just look at our approach to travel safety. There's probably not one person who doesn't think about this. You wear a seatbelt, obey traffic laws, and yield to pedestrians. But life-saving vitality behavior safety is often an afterthought.

The Sustaining Tool for Recharging the Business of Wellbeing

An organization can't survive without the executives who run things. The success and wellbeing of the executives and the business go hand in hand. When advising leaders on performance and business success, sustaining vitality and wellbeing must be included. There's no magic pill that can recharge energy and output. However, I'm happy to tell you that researchers are discovering simple, everyday actions you can take to create the vigor and gusto needed to *be well, do well, and flourish*. It starts with appreciating the importance of the supporting tools of sustainable vitality behaviors to recharge the business of wellbeing.

SIX SUPPORTING VITALITY BEHAVIORS OF RECHARGING THE BUSINESS OF WELLBEING

1. *Optimized sleep hygiene*

In a conversation with Pam, CEO of a marketing firm, she admitted to sleeping five to six hours a night, feeling it's enough. She assumed that one or two fewer hours of sleep wouldn't affect how she felt the following day. Pam believed she was performing quite well and said to us, "We used to do this in college when studying for exams, and that turned out all right." At our insistence, she agreed to experiment with going to bed a couple of hours earlier to see how she felt the following day.

To her amazement, Pam told us she was more attuned to her environment and her emotions and was able to recognize the emotions of others. I can attest to this. Many nights I would lay awake and sleep only about three to four hours if that. It was horrible. But now, with a full eight hours of sleep each night, my creativity and mental acuity are greatly enhanced. I feel like a different person, full of vitality, zest, and the capacity to remain focused on my work.

CHAPTER 12: Recharging The Business Of Wellbeing: Conscious Leadership

Like Pam, you may be accustomed to five or six hours of sleep. What you may not realize is studies show this subtle behavior damages your health, cognitive capacity, and mood and hijacks your wellbeing and performance. One study found that losing as little as ninety minutes of sleep reduces our daytime alertness by nearly one-third.[5] And studies by another researcher found that four hours of sleep loss will produce as much impairment as consuming a six-pack, and a whole night of sleep loss is equivalent to having a blood alcohol content of 0.19.[6] Not only does lack of sleep affect mood and concentration in the short term, but over time, it increases the risks of developing Alzheimer's disease, diabetes, and certain cancers.[7]

Here's what you need to do:

The challenge with sleep deprivation is that we get accustomed to performing sub-optimally. Sleep is the key to optimizing vitality and achieving high performance. Prioritizing sufficient sleep and rest enables your mind and body to recharge and perform at their best.

   a. Avoid big meals late in the evening. Eat earlier.
   b. Avoid caffeine after midday. Caffeine found in coffee, tea, and even chocolate can make it more difficult to get to sleep and stay asleep.
   c. Avoid late-night exercise. Don't exercise for three hours before going to sleep.
   d. Reduce alcohol consumption. Alcohol harms our sleep quality.
   e. Avoid phones, tablets, and TV immediately before bed. The light from these digital sources can overstimulate your brain and interrupt your sleep. (Adapted from National Institute on Aging)

To improve sleep quality, you also need to reduce worry and stress. Research by psychologist Martin Seligman shows that gratitude can increase wellbeing and help with sleep. Seligman advocates writing three good things or three blessings every night before going to bed, which allows you to turn your attention to the positive. Here's how this looks:

a. Set aside 10 minutes every night before you go to bed to think about a positive event or thing that happened to you that day.
b. Write down these three positive things.
c. Reflect on why each good thing happened. Then write your answer next to the event.

2. *Optimized physical activity*

I get my best ideas during my morning walks. Steve Jobs was known for his walking meetings. Harry S. Truman woke up at 5:00 a.m. for a vigorous walk wearing a business suit and tie. Sigmund Freud conducted walking consultations and evaluations. I've observed my husband pacing back and forth on occasion when in deep thought. Stanford researchers Marily Oppezzo and Daniel L. Schwartz provide an explanation for this:

"People have noted that walking seems to have a special relation to creativity. Four studies demonstrate that walking increases creative ideation. The effect is not simply due to the increased perceptual stimulation of moving through an environment, but rather it is due to walking. Whether one is outdoors or on a treadmill, walking improves the generation of novel yet appropriate ideas, and the effect even extends to when people sit down to do their creative work shortly after. Walking opens up the free flow of ideas, and it is a simple and robust solution to the goals of increasing creativity and increasing physical activity."[8]

As you can see, any physical activity is a good antidote to a sedentary workday and beneficial to sustaining vitality behaviors and wellbeing. According to Robert Gotlin, DO, a specialist in sports medicine at Lenox Hill and Mt. Sinai Hospitals in New York City, the benefits of exercise for your energy level are twofold: Exercise boosts your body's fitness and your mood, both of which contribute to your overall health and wellbeing.

You'd be amazed by the hours you spend sitting at work. On average, many people are sitting nine to ten hours a day. Think about that. It's more time than many people spend sleeping. I enjoy an hour's walk in the mornings before I start my workday, along with some moderate weight training at the gym and occasionally evening bike rides with my husband. This works for us, and you can tailor your activities and schedules to what works best for you. The key is to move more and sit less to recharge your vitality. If you're new to physical activity (I hope you aren't), start by discussing this with your doctor and trying different things to learn which physical activities you enjoy most.

Here's what you need to know:

- a. Build smart habits like taking the stairs instead of the elevator, moving every twenty minutes away from sitting at your desk, and walking to the refrigerator for a drink instead of asking your spouse or children to bring one to you. You've heard this before but it's worth repeating.

- b. Physical activity, like regular exercise, recharges many areas of your performance wellbeing. Researchers suggest 150 minutes (2.5 hours) of heart-pumping physical activity and being active at least 300 minutes (5 hours) per week.[9]

- c. Boost your activity level by walking or jogging, stretching, lifting weights, or walking on the treadmill either at home or the gym while watching your must-see TV shows.

- d. My neighbor breaks it up into 10 to 15 minutes a few times a day to get his workout activity in. We often catch him walking around the community, pulling himself up by a tree bough, jogging, or riding his bike.

3. *Optimized nutrition*

We've all experienced that mid-afternoon crash, somewhere between lunch and dinner, when your attention wanes, your motivation fades, and you're feeling like napping. You can avoid the midday slump with the right nutrition.

There's an overabundance of advice on what we should or shouldn't eat or drink. Should I count calories, carbohydrates, or fats? Is breakfast truly the most important meal of the day, or is it fine to try intermittent fasting? You will get conflicting responses from different sources. However, I believe we can all agree that it's best not to consume certain foods and drinks regularly that are detrimental to our health and wellbeing.

You need awareness. An awareness of what enables your body to function optimally in certain areas, including disease prevention, energy production, immunity, and physical and mental performance, starts with nutrition. But here's the problem. We generally think of food only in terms of calories, but in fact, it's the proper nutrition that keeps your energy levels high.

Here's what you need to know:

a. Food has a direct impact on your cognitive performance, which is why a poor decision about what you eat for lunch can derail an entire afternoon.

b. Our bodies process different foods at different rates. For example, some foods, like pasta, bread, cereal, and soda, release their glucose quickly, leading to a burst of energy, but are then followed by a slump.[10] I intentionally avoid these foods.

c. Cardiac surgeon Dr. Philip Ovadia encourages us to eat as many real whole foods as possible. This gives us a much wider range of nutrition instead of dumping in a bunch of calories.[11]

d. By eating smart, avoiding high-carb foods, sugar, and eating good meats, sometimes leafy vegetables, and berries (along with a regular exercise routine), I lost 10 pounds within two months, which enables

CHAPTER 12: Recharging The Business Of Wellbeing: Conscious Leadership

me to keep my energy high. I can guarantee that these results weighed strongly on my nutritional intake. Learning to understand the foods I eat and how my body works with these foods was my launching pad toward metabolic health, more energy, and vitality. To learn more on this subject, I highly recommend that you read Dr. Philip Ovadia's book: *Stay Off My Operating Table*.

e. The foods we consume have a profound impact on our vitality. If you've been a bit sluggish at work, I recommend recharging the business of wellbeing with healthy nutritional habits, including real superfoods like beef, salmon, eggs, avocados, berries, and nuts. Because we're unique, there's no single nutrition plan that works for everyone. Find what works for you, and don't put it off into the future. No, it isn't always easy, but you have authority over your *fighting-ego* when it tries to derail you.

4. *Optimized mental energy*

I operate my company from my home on a full business schedule, and for many years, I suffered significant exhaustion at the end of the day. Thinking that my exhaustion was caused by busyness, I discovered it had more to do with being mentally fatigued. It sounds strange to say, but on some days, my brain was tired. Researchers refer to mental fatigue as a psychobiological state caused by prolonged periods of demanding cognitive activity. That's a fancy way of saying we have too many decisions, too much work, too many interruptions, demands, and shifts in attention without time to pause and recharge.[12]

Like me, you probably didn't realize how mental exhaustion impacts your behavior as well as brings on physical and emotional symptoms. For example, it was out of character for me to withdraw socially and cancel appointments, even virtual appointments, but I had started to do this. I noticed that even though I wanted to complete my tasks, for a while, it became difficult to concentrate on any one assignment, so I caught myself multitasking. We know from Chapter 5 that multitasking is a productivity illusion. But the worst was having brain fog kick in, causing me to become short-tempered and irritated more easily than normal. Physically, extra pounds appeared, and I suffered many sleepless nights. I knew then I needed to find ways for some self-care to recharge my wellbeing.

Here's what you need to know:

a. It's interesting to me now that I would drop everything and take a long brisk walk to recharge and energize my thinking. Several studies show the value of this for boosting concentration and mental focus.[13] Staying close to nature improves physical, mental, and spiritual wellbeing and makes us feel alive from the inside.

b. Mental wellbeing is an important contributor to business productivity, success, and job satisfaction.[14]

c. Hours are fixed. Energy is not. Shifting from time management to energy management helps you to become more conscious and intentional about managing your energy. Track your energy levels. Create a log and track your energy levels throughout the entire day. Note what you're doing at hourly intervals from 7:00 a.m. until 10:00 p.m. using the following scale for measuring your energy levels: 1-2: very low; 3-4: low; 5-6: neutral; 7-8: high; 9-10: very high.

d. Evaluate your energy level patterns. At what times was your energy high? At what times was your energy low? What patterns can you observe about the activities associated with high energy? What patterns can you observe about the activities linked to low energy?

CHAPTER 12: Recharging The Business Of Wellbeing: Conscious Leadership

e. Replenish your energy resources. Energy can be managed physically by building endurance and fitness; mentally by cultivating focus and attention; emotionally by cultivating excitement and connection; and spiritually by cultivating presence. Observing what you're doing when your energy is high during your day can help you to come up with possible energy-boosting actions when at your lowest.

f. Remove yourself from work mentally. When your working hours end, distance yourself psychologically. Don't take work home with you or work on projects during your time off. Be conscious of improving your ability to manage your daily routines, your work, and your social relationships to maintain a positive energy balance and improve your vitality.

5. *Optimized prayer and meditation*

In Chapter 2, I shared with you the genesis of *Lead2Flourish* and, subsequently, this book. It came to me while I was in prayer. I can't emphasize enough the importance of having morning meditation time before beginning your day. I believe it's a surefire component of your performance and business of wellbeing. Chief Justice Clarence Thomas said, "I go to mass before I go to work. The reason for that is not just habit. It gives you a centering ... starts you on a way of doing a secular job the right way for the right reasons."

Regardless of personal faith, belief, or intention, prayer and meditation affect our behavior. Dr. David Spiegel at Stanford University School of Medicine says, "Prayer and meditation are highly effective in lowering our reactivity to traumatic and negative events. Praying involves the deeper parts of the brain, and these parts of the brain are involved in self-reflection and self-soothing. Studies also show that prayer reduces anxiety and depression. An anxiety reduction allows people to process and react to external events more cognitively rather than emotionally.[15]

Here's what you need to know:

a. Praying and meditation removes the focus from you and your specific task.

b. Praying and meditation channel spiritual energy throughout your brain.

c. The first twenty minutes of your day are crucial to the attitude of the rest of the day. Prayer and meditation vitalize you to start it off right, giving you the potential to have a great day every day.

d. According to Dr. Loretta G. Breuning, author of *The Science of Positivity* and *Habits of a Happy Brain*, "All too often, we rush through our day and overlook our deeper impulses. Then when our work is done, and we try to rest, the bad feelings we've ignored surge up, and we have trouble untangling the cause and finding a solution that restores hope. Praying makes that useful conscious act into a reliable habit."

e. Psychotherapist Dr. Paul Hokemeyer adds, "One of the purposes of prayer and meditation is to regain our footing so that we can step out into the world and take positive action: we reconnect, re-center, recharge, and gain the strength necessary to take steps that will create real change. In other words, prayer is the fuel that lights the fire of action."

6. *Optimized conscious speaking*

I bet you didn't see this coming, did you? Your words contribute to performance and wellbeing and are just as important to you as exercise and good nutrition. And words are so powerful that they created the universe. The force of power behind God's words at the creation, "Let there be light," crystalized the behavior of matter, and there was light! Today, the phrase "words create worlds" is often used by psychology practitioners whose work

CHAPTER 12: Recharging The Business Of Wellbeing: Conscious Leadership

highlights the importance of language and conversation in coaching, therapy, and consulting. How we speak shapes our beliefs and drive our behaviors. In their book, *Words Can Change Your Brain*, Andrew Newberg, MD, and Mark Robert Waldman say, "A single word has the power to influence the expression of genes that regulate physical and emotional stress."[16] Don't allow your *fighting-ego* to get in the way of purposeful communication.

When I worked in corporate, I was expected to work and live by my word. When I made a promise to do something, I had to do it. If I broke my word and didn't carry out the responsibilities expected of me, it negatively impacted the team's performance and my vitality. The tunes of excuses that played over and over in my head sounded like, "The train was running late?" or "Can I get this right just once?" Your *fighting-ego* will throw out every excuse imaginable when you break a promise. We are programmed to accept this as normal.

Are you conscious of what you say? Do you throw words without first thinking about what you're saying? Unfortunately, this zaps your business performance, wellbeing, and vitality. Words are seeds that are planted into the atmosphere when you speak. Where you are now, how you perform, and what you're experiencing is tied to word seeds that you've planted (spoken) before.

Here's what you need to know:

a. Words, spoken, written, or even used in internal dialogue, can influence how others feel about you and how you feel about yourself. What damage do you create with unconscious behavior patterns of criticizing and berating yourself or others?

b. You don't see the harmful results of your word choices in tangible ways. It can be challenging to be conscious of their consequences, especially when words are directed at you.

c. Do you ever say, "My work is stressful," "I feel overwhelmed," or "I can't do this"? Unconscious, unhelpful speech can land you where you'd never imagined being.

d. Change starts with you. You need to change your beliefs about your or others' abilities before you can change your words.
e. Your words are the tools with which you create your world. Listen to your thoughts and ask yourself, "Do I need to say this? Do I truly mean what I say? Will what I say hurt or help me and someone else?" Then you should consciously choose the best words to create your best world.
f. Not only do words create your world, but also the world of others.

Certainly, the business of wellbeing starts at the top. There's a direct correlation between team performance and the wellbeing awareness of its leader.

Lead2Flourish Keys

1. Performance is about wellbeing. Optimizing wellbeing is about behavior.
2. Behavior, wellbeing, performance, and business success are not mutually exclusive.
3. As we are conditioned in our behaviors, then wellbeing and health take on a different posture.
4. Performance wellbeing is the process of tapping into desired behaviors that enables us to *be well, do well, and flourish* in business and life.
5. Subtle behavior patterns may seem innocent and insignificant but can hijack our efforts to be well and do well. We generally brush them aside because our *fighting-egos* have convinced us this is who we are and how we're wired.
6. The business of wellbeing must be central to any business strategy. The success and wellbeing of the executives and the business go hand in hand.
7. Researchers are discovering simple, everyday actions you can take to create the vigor and gusto needed to *be well, do well, and flourish* by

optimizing sleep hygiene, physical activity, good nutrition, mental energy, and conscious speaking.

Questions for Reflection

1. What can you do now to improve your wellbeing and increase your vitality?
2. What can you do to improve the quality of your sleep hygiene?
3. How will you trim down a sedentary workday to upgrade vitality behaviors and wellbeing?
4. What nutritional guidelines will you adopt for achieving more vitality?
5. What are your intrinsic motivators for more mental energy and conscious speaking?

Designing a Lead2Flourish Plan – Recharging the Business of Wellbeing

Reflecting on what you've learned in this chapter, design your plan for enhancing your vitality and recharging the business of wellbeing.

1. The subtle behaviors I'm facing are:
2. I've decided to commit to:
3. The reasons I've made this decision are:
4. Potential *fighting-ego* hurdles:
5. How can I intentionally recharge through sleep hygiene, physical activity, good nutrition, mental energy, and conscious speaking?
6. This is how I will introduce recharging the business of wellbeing to my organization:
7. I will help my people with understanding the business of wellbeing and the tools to flourish by:
8. My timeline:

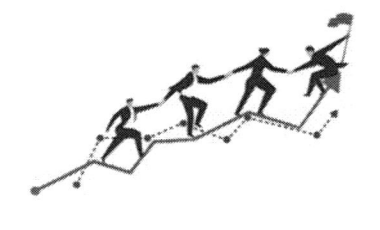

CHAPTER 13

RECHARGING WITH GRATITUDE: SUPPORTIVE LEADERSHIP

The Remarkable Mr. Mulley

When I began my corporate career, Mr. Mulley was my boss. Mr. Mulley was a remarkable executive, probably one of the best I've ever met. His love for his work and desire to inspire his employees were widely noticeable. He knew how to take the risk out of confrontation by attacking issues in a way that didn't make people the victim. His difficult conversations weren't difficult. It was easy to talk honestly and openly about real issues and how to support others without struggle.

As I advanced in my career with other companies, I often thought about Mr. Mulley and wondered why it seemed so easy for him but hard for others to enhance people's level of engagement and commitment. I believe the difference was how he acknowledged people in an authentic and heartfelt manner by always guiding his conversations and actions with the art of gratitude.

Ralph Waldo Emerson shared this insight on the art of gratitude: "Cultivate the habit of being grateful for every good thing that comes to you and to give thanks continuously. And because all things have contributed to your advancement, you should include all things in your gratitude."

Studies support my far-reaching experiences in leadership mastery (acknowledgment, appreciation, and gratitude are all conscious behaviors and part of my leadership model). Douglas R. Conant, former President and CEO of Campbell Soup Company, demonstrated this well. He handwrote over 30,000 thank you cards to his employees, from maintenance people to senior executives. His dedication to "tough-minded performance standards with tender-heartedness" led to an engaged workforce and financial salvation during the Great Recession.

"Handwritten notes may seem like a waste of time," writes Conant, "but in my experience, they build goodwill and lead to higher productivity."[1] No doubt, gestures like this are what motivate people to do their best work, knowing that it matters to someone.

Unfortunately, as I write this book, there are challenges everywhere in our professional and personal lives, namely COVID-19, rising inflation, and emerging tyranny in world government. It seems to have affected some more than others. Many have linked COVID-19 to a phenomenon labeled "the great resignation" whereby people are voluntarily leaving the workplace in massive numbers. These challenges have prompted a time when people are evaluating their sense of meaning in life, including what work means to them.

In these COVID times and beyond, leaders must honestly assess how well people are accomplishing work responsibilities. This is done by recognizing their strengths and contributions and valuing them using expressions of gratitude as the highlighter. According to Massachusetts-based talent management company Workhuman, "With just five moments of recognition

CHAPTER 13: Recharging With Gratitude: Supportive Leadership

per year (that's less than one 'thank you' every two months), voluntary turnover is reduced by 22%."[2] The most powerful accessory in your inventory when it comes to keeping and attracting talent is gratitude.

Gratitude tops my list of ways to recharge. There are numerous physical, social, and emotional benefits of gratitude. Professor researcher Robert Emmons has authored several papers on the psychology of gratitude, showing that being more grateful can lead to increased levels of wellbeing.[3]

In his book, *Thanks! How the New Science of Gratitude Can Make You Happier*, suggests that you integrate gratitude into your daily life rather than make it something you need to add to an already busy day. He defines gratitude as the ability to recognize the goodness in your life. Emmons says gratitude is a relationship-strengthening emotion because it requires people to see how they've been supported and affirmed by others.

The Most Attractive Leadership Accessory

When referring to leadership traits, we generally think of words such as confident, passionate, creative, and focused. While studying this topic, I didn't find gratitude listed as a leadership trait. I guess it appears awkward to recognize it as such. Perhaps it doesn't fit the depiction for some, but it should. However, to clarify, the research of McCullough, Emmons, and Tsang did find gratitude as being a trait—shown by an individual who practices gratitude as part of their daily life.[4] In contrast, the research of Watkins, Van Gelder, and Frias discovered gratitude as being a state—the rich emotion experienced by a person when someone expresses gratitude for them.[5] These studies conclude then that gratitude is both a trait and a state, and is an attractive leadership accessory.

It was easy to recognize these accessories on Mr. Mulley. He effortlessly extended and received gratitude and didn't cave to his *fighting-ego*. When someone didn't perform to his standards, instead of reacting harshly, Mr. Mulley often said, "Let's find a way to make this work better for everyone." We worked on projects together as a team where everyone was required to equally contribute knowledge and expertise.

During one instance, there was a new hire who, from my perspective, wasn't seasoned enough in how we did things. I could see by his awkwardness he wasn't comfortable, yet he tried to fit in. To be honest, his mistakes outnumbered his contributions. During one of our morning exploratory sessions, Mr. Mulley mentioned how each of us had specifically contributed to the project and took time to make sure we felt seen and appreciated. And he didn't leave out the new hire as he received the same recognition as everyone else.

Although Mr. Mulley could've taken the new hire's performance personally as reflecting poorly on him as a leader, he didn't, even though it was a serious ego threat to his reputation. The fact that he responded with positive recognition and gratitude confirmed Emmons' theory for me, namely that gratitude is a relationship-strengthening emotion because it requires people to see how they've been supported and affirmed by others. Mr. Mulley showed that he was grateful for the new hire, not merely the performance.

Gratitude is not simply being thankful when things go well. It entails recognizing that we have an understanding that our experiences have meaning and value even when things go wrong. This is a key flourishing attitude, and it's proven in research that Mr. Mulley's gratitude expressions increased his prosocial behavior by enabling all of us to feel socially valued.[6]

Unfortunately, many success-driven leaders underuse their powerful gratitude accessory to appreciate the unique contributions of their people. One *Forbes* writer wrote, "Feeling grateful can make you more successful."[7] Bersin and Associates confirm this success factor in their study, revealing companies that "excel at employee recognition" are twelve times more likely to enjoy strong business results.[8]

From studying this topic and my years of working with leaders, I have categorized six behavior shifts when you are grateful.

CHAPTER 13: Recharging With Gratitude: Supportive Leadership

Six Gratitude Behavior Shifts

1. Gratitude Behavior Shift 1: From Difficult Focus to Strength Focus

   Grateful leaders are more likely to focus on their strengths and move away from focusing on difficulties. Stress-resilience increases as a result, which aids in better handling anxiety when faced with adversity and trauma.

2. Gratitude Behavior Shift 2: From Selfish Focus to Selfless Focus

   When leaders are grateful, they are likely to want to improve their relationships with others in general and within organizations and groups. Leaders and others are recharged by this.

3. Grateful Behavior Shift 3: From Carefree Focus to What Matters Focus

   Grateful leaders are more likely to focus on personal and organizational growth and less likely to engage in unhelpful ego drivers, such as envy, resentment, greed, and bitterness. As a result, they recharge themselves and others to give their best work.

4. Grateful Behavior Shift 4: From Workplace Blahs to Workplace Satisfaction

   A leader's attitude of gratitude can recharge the environment, where trust is established, a sense of community is built, and work-related stress is decreased.

5. Grateful Behavior Shift 5: From Social Alienation to Social Bonding

   Leaders who feel grateful and encourage gratitude in the workplace are likely to reap the benefits of stronger group cohesiveness and an engaged workforce. Because gratitude is a many-sided social emotion, it can bring people together in pursuit of a greater vision.

6. Grateful Behavior Shift 6: From Reserved to Recharged

   Gratitude helps leaders to be compassionate, considerate, empathetic, and loved, among others. With these traits, leaders recognize good work, give everyone their due importance in the group, and actively communicate with the team members.

Narrowing the Gratitude Gap

Zig Ziglar said, "Gratitude is the healthiest of all human emotions." I agree with Ziglar. So, despite the compelling benefits, why doesn't it happen in the workplace? According to a Harris Interactive survey on behalf of Glassdoor, seven in ten (68%) employees say their boss shows them enough appreciation; however, more than half (53%) of employees admit they would stay longer at their company if they felt more appreciation from their boss. Four in five (81%) employees report they're motivated to work harder when their boss shows appreciation for their work, higher than the 38% of employees who say they're motivated to work harder when their boss is demanding, or the 37% of employees who say they're motivated to work harder because they fear losing their job.[9]

Wharton Professor Adam Grant believes a gratitude gap occurs because people don't like to admit they need help at work, and thanking someone means admitting you couldn't do it all on your own.[10] This, to me, sounds like a *fighting-ego* is controlling the situation. I believe psychologists Shai Davidai and Thomas Gilovich have the answer to closing the gap. They believe we tend to focus more on the obstacles and difficulties of life because they demand some action. We have to fight and overcome them to get back to the normal flow of life.

(Remember what we said in Chapter 9 about leaders often studying and trying to fix the weaknesses—what went wrong or what's broken?) Davidai and Gilovich go on to say, on the flip side, we forget to attend to the better things in life because they're already there (like believing your employees will be there every day), and we don't have to do anything (like showing gratitude) to make them stay with us. Practicing gratitude, according to Gilovich, is the best way to remind ourselves of the things that give us the courage to move on in life (thus, a way to close the gratitude gap).[11]

FIVE PRINCIPLES OF RECHARGING WITH GRATITUDE

While gratitude is a basic human emotion, ungratefulness has been described as the solvent of social bonds and an assault on flourishing human life.[12] In a time when chronic stress and workplace burnout are at an all-time high, one of the most powerful ways to rewire your brain and recharge for more joy and less anxiety is to focus on gratitude. These five principles will edge you onward:

1. *Savor the good*

Shift your focus from what's not working at work and in life to the good that is working. Emmons believes, through our senses, we gain an appreciation of what it means to be human and of what an incredible miracle it is to be alive. That's what "good" looks like. Seen through the lens of gratitude, the human body is not only a miraculous construction but also a gift.

Here's what you need to do:

Establish a smart habit of reflecting on the good aspects of your work for which you're grateful, including the people you work with. Reflect on being grateful for your job, business, your supportive work relationships, and the sacrifices or contributions that others have made for you. According to research, this can boost your gratitude levels.[13] Robert Brault said, "Enjoy the little things, for one day you may look back and realize they were the big things."

2. *Don't fake it, feel it*

Accept that you may initially feel uncomfortable if you aren't accustomed to expressing gratitude. But you don't need to fake it. Think about a time when someone said thank you, and you knew it was ingenuine. How did it make you feel? People can tell when an expression of thanks is not genuine.

Here's what you need to do:

Using the subtraction method, take a moment to reflect on how you rely on the contributions of those around you. Think about one individual in particular whose contributions stand out. Now imagine if this person was not part of your team. What would be lost? Think about these things when you extend your gratitude. You'll feel it and not need to fake it. Albert Schweitzer said, "At times, our own light goes out and is rekindled by a spark from another person. Each of us has cause to think with deep gratitude of those who have lighted the flame within us."

3. Be distinctive, specific, and people-centric

If your leader arbitrarily showed gratitude to the entire team with a general "great job," how would you know if he or she was thinking of your contributions? Remember, a general notion of gratitude can apply to anyone. So be specific when showing your humanity.

Here's what you need to do:

Determine in what specific ways the individual has contributed to the team and company. Acknowledge what the individual did. Your extension of gratitude is more genuine if you mention specifically what the person did rather than the outcomes and results of what they did. Outcomes could have resulted from factors beyond any one individual's control. William Arthur Ward said, "Feeling gratitude and not expressing it is like wrapping a present and not giving it."

CHAPTER 13: Recharging With Gratitude: Supportive Leadership

4. Embrace the golden rule

As children, we're taught to do unto others as we would have them do unto us. This mantra can serve you well in your day-to-day expressions of gratitude. People see us by our behaviors.

Here's what you need to do:

Our behaviors and actions provide another avenue for the expression of gratitude. Be respectful and treat others with the level of courtesy you would like to receive. Smile, be patient, listen and express kindness whenever possible. Bring drinks for your colleagues the next time you visit the coffee bar. Show that you value them. Henri Frederic Amiel said, "Thankfulness may consist merely of words. Gratitude is shown in acts."

5. Vow and commit to practicing gratitude

Research shows that making an oath to perform a behavior increases the likelihood that the action will be executed. You may not only reap the rewards in terms of promoting a positive mental state while reducing negativity but also get into the habit of focusing on the positive—in time, it can become second nature. Place sticky notes where you can see them as a reminder. Visual reminders like this can serve as cues to trigger gratitude thoughts.

Here's what you need to do:

Write your gratitude vow, which could be as simple as "I vow to acknowledge the good I see every day." Post it somewhere where you will be reminded of it every day. The next time someone does something you appreciate, challenge yourself to let them know. Melody Beattie said, "Gratitude turns what we have into enough and more. It turns denial into acceptance, chaos into order, confusion into clarity ... it makes sense of our past, brings peace for today, and creates a vision for tomorrow."

Something to Consider Going Forward

Supportive leadership comes with positive results. Grateful leaders and those who receive gratitude are likely to experience greater psychological, spiritual, and physical wellbeing. Taking others for granted and what they contribute, be it large or small, cancels out the goodness we have within us.

In his TED talk, David Steindl-Rast offers practical advice for recharging with gratitude based on the advice to children when learning to cross the road:

STOP: We rush through life and miss opportunities because we don't stop to recognize and act on them.

LOOK: We must use all our senses to enjoy the richness that life has given to us.

GO: We should do whatever life offers to us in that present moment. Sometimes that might be difficult, but we should go with it and do our best to enjoy every moment.[14]

Lead2Flourish Keys

1. Acknowledgment, appreciation, and gratitude are conscious behaviors and part of the leadership model.
2. Gratitude motivates people to do their best work, knowing that it matters to someone and can lead to increased levels of wellbeing.
3. Professor Robert Emmons says gratitude is a relationship-strengthening emotion because it requires people to see how they've been supported and affirmed by others.
4. Gratitude is the most powerful accessory a leader can wear.
5. Research shows four in five (81%) employees report they're motivated to work harder when their boss shows appreciation for their work.

6. One of the most powerful ways to rewire your brain for more joy and less stress is to focus on gratitude.

Questions for Reflection

1. Think of a time when someone expressed their appreciation for you. What emotions did you experience? Take 60 seconds to feel your gratitude.
2. Take some time to think about the things around you that make you feel grateful. What are you grateful for? Who are you grateful for? Why?
3. What experience are you grateful for? What challenge are you grateful for? Why?
4. Take a moment to consider your employees, partners, and colleagues. What makes you feel grateful to have them in your life?
5. Why do you want to express and receive gratitude? How has it positively impacted you?

Designing a Lead2Flourish Plan – Recharging with Gratitude

Reflecting on what you learned in this chapter, design a plan to become recharged with gratitude to reduce negativity and promote a positive mental state.

1. I've avoided the behavior of expressing gratitude at work because:
2. I've decided to commit to:
3. The reasons I've made this decision are:
4. Potential *fighting-ego* hurdles:
5. I will intentionally close any gratitude gaps in the workplace and my life in these ways:

6. I will introduce recharging gratitude to my organization and turn it into a competitive advantage to be an embedded part of the company's culture by:
7. My timeline:

FINAL THOUGHTS

THE ESSENCE TO ENDURE

My Wish for You

One purpose of *Lead2Flourish* is to provide insight into the costs of your unhelpful behaviors and introduce resources to help you become a more conscious and efficient leader. But my wish for you is more than that. My wish is that you've also learned to create a context that empowers others. And the sum of what I wish for you is to trust yourself. It's said that it's easier to trust others than to trust yourself. I'm betting on you and inviting you to come along with me and bet on yourself.

The *Lead2Flourish* skillset is my core message. Going forward, I want you to understand how leadership is both an art and a science: the art of recognizing and uncovering specific ego-protected patterns—searching for the ego threats that drive unhelpful behaviors and then realizing the costs to yourself, your relationships, your organization, and your community; the science of conscious choice—the decision to support your performance wellbeing and build a more honest and productive environment around you from the inspiration within you to flourish.

Imagine an alliance of flourishing leaders whose flourishing minds, attitudes, thought processes, and lives understand the same resources and share the same commitment to empowering others to feel noticed, affirmed, and needed. I hope you're better equipped to deal with the human and emotional aspects of your work. I hope that you will welcome constructive feedback and confront issues head-on. I hope that you are challenged to support your team and your company rather than satisfy your ego. I hope that you have an open, undefended dialogue and are willing to stand up and be vulnerable.

When leaders can look at themselves to see who they are and how that determines their actions and their paths, it can accelerate an organization's progress and a community's evolution. My wish is that you've recognized and retired your *fighting-ego syndrome*, first by developing the awareness to break through those unconscious habits and behaviors, second by taking the risk to behave differently, third by repeatedly practicing the new behavior, and fourth by designing a new path for achieving results in line with your important goals.

My wish for you is that the renovation of your outdated ways of thinking has enlivened the power and harmony of your vision, values, and voice to guide strategies. My wish for you is to be defined by your best strengths, fueled by your emotional resilience, recharged by your business of wellbeing, and preserved by your gratitude. My wish for you is that your new awareness shifts your company into higher gear. My wish for you is that *Lead2Flourish* becomes the culture.

I hope you experience the same joy and excitement in implementing the principles in this book as I have had in sharing them with you. My wish is that you lead with self-awareness, accountability, agility, integrity, and

FINAL THOUGHTS: The Essence To Endure

authenticity and model this capability to others. I wish for you to recognize and accept this work as the much-needed enhancement that fills the deficit in leadership development approaches you've experienced.

The genuine in you know that the time is ripe to commit and make your wellbeing a priority. The genuine in you know it's time to commit to moving from the end of strings that something else pulls. You now have the right tools to turn this commitment into impact. My wish for you is that the *fighting-ego syndrome* will no longer pull your strings, but through the pages of this book, you'll be led by the genuine in you. For genuineness energizes you to *Lead2Flourish*.

Let's Stay Connected

Reach out to me at DrDeana.com for my workshops, consulting, coaching, and speaking. Follow me on Twitter, LinkedIn @DrDeanaMurphy, and on Instagram @dr_DeanaMurphy.

At any time you can revisit the *www.DrDeana.com/assessment* page to learn where you are on the *Flourishing IQ* scale.

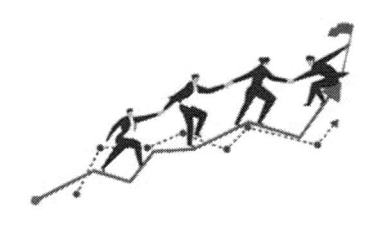

ACKNOWLEDGMENTS

I'm very grateful

Writing a book can be a long and lonely quest. Early mornings and late nights I began putting my thoughts on paper, tossing ideas around in hopes it all made sense. And then the world seemed to stop because of COVID. While attending a Zoom meeting someone told us to not write a book but to use the time and energy for creating income-producing ideas. While this was good advice, I'm very grateful for writing this book and being a part of your journey.

To my best friend, confidant, life partner, and amazing husband, Eric. Your support, encouragement, and belief in my vision have allowed me to complete another book and keep reaching higher.

To my editors Daniel DeCillis and Hayley Sherman, and my proofreader Liz Saucedo who helped me to make *Lead2Flourish* come alive on the page.

To Joshua Lisec, who showed me how to convey the spirit and solutions of *Lead2Flourish* in a simple, inspiring, and captivating subtitle.

To my clients, who have entrusted me with their life experiences, you did the real work. I'm grateful for the opportunity to work with you.

NOTES

Chapter 1. Introduction: The Essence to Flourish

1. Smithsonian Magazine (November 10, 2015), "When the Empire State Building Was Just an Architect's Sketch"
2. https://prabook.com/web/william.lamb/3759143
3. (2014) The Associated Schools of Construction, "Analyzing the Empire State Building Project from the Perspective of Lean Project Delivery System", retrieved from http://ascpro0.ascweb.org/archives/cd/2014/paper/CPGT267002014.pdf
4. The Empire State Building: Construction, History and Facts, Parker, Waichman, LLP, Retrieved from https://www.yourlawyer.com/library/empire-state-building-history/
5. Originally published in the Art Deco New York journal, Vol. 1, Issue 1, Spring 2016, Retrieved from https://www.artdeco.org/empire-state-building-interview
6. Gallup Workplace Report, Retrieved from https://www.gallup.com/workplace/352949/employee-engagement-holds-steady-first-half-2021.aspx
7. https://www.willistowerswatson.com/en-US/Solutions/future-of-work
8. Hoffman and Smits, "Cognitive Behavior Therapy" www.ncbi.nlm.nih.gov/pmc/articles/PMC2409267
9. https://emersus.com/services/executive-effectiveness-suite/executive-personal-problem-resolution/
   https://libraryofprofessionalcoaching.com/concepts/managing-stress-and-challenges/ignoring-the-personal-stress-of-a-key-executive-could-cost-you-millions/17/
10. https://www.bupaglobal.com/en/your-wellbeing/our-research/wellbeing-index-2021

LEAD2FLOURISH

Chapter 2. Lead2Flourish

1. How to Shift From Languishing to Flourishing: Q&A with Adam Grant. Retrieved from https://blog.asana.com/2021/07/languishing-flourishing/#close
2. Retrieved from Why Leadership Development Programs Fail, https://www.mckinsey.com/featured-insights/leadership/why-leadership-development-programs-fail
3. Viktor Frankl, Man's Search for Meaning, Beacon Press, (January 1, 1746).
4. http://sonjalyubomirsky.com/wp-content/themes/sonjalyubomirsky/papers/LSS2005.pdf

Chapter 3. Unconscious Gaps & Recognizing Root Causes

1. https://psychologenie.com/aaron-beck-cognitive-behavior-theory
2. https://www.reuters.com/article/us-global-race-wells-fargo-exclusive-idUSKCN26D2IU and https://www.foxbusiness.com/markets/wells-fargo-ceo-charlie-scharf-diversity-limited-black-talent-apology
3. Baumeister, R., Bratslavsky, E, Finkenaur, C., & Vohs, K.D. "Bad is Stronger than Good." Review of General Psychology, 5, 4, 323-370., 2001
4. Yale University, Adverse Childhood Experiences and Their Influence On Social Connectedness, Tammie Kwong, elischolar.library.yale.edu/cgi/viewcontent.cgi?referer=&httpsredir=1&article=1156&context=ysphtdl https://txicfw.socialwork.utexas.edu/adverse-childhood-experiences-aces-study/
5. Donna Jackson Nakazawa, Childhood Disrupted: How Your Biography Becomes Your Biology, and How You Can Heal, Atria Books; (July 7, 2015)

Chapter 4. Recognizing the Traps & the Liabilities

1. https://www.pearsonassessments.com/professional-assessments/products/authors/beck-aaron.html
2. Dr. Caroline Leaf, "Switch On Your Brain", Baker Books, Michigan, 2013.
3. Dr. Caroline Leaf, "Who Switched Off My Brain", Baker Books, Michigan, 2013.
4. Ibid
5. http://shawnetv.com/
6. https://news.yale.edu/2018/09/17/we-are-predisposed-forgive-new-research-suggests
7. Sanjay, Singh, R., & Hooda, R. S. (2019). Forgiveness: A theoretical perspective. IAHRW International Journal of Social Sciences Review, 7(4), 687–689.

Chapter 5. Myths & Misinformation: Recognizing the Damages

Behavior Myth #1 – Overthinking is Problem Solving

1. https://www.nature.com/articles/s41598-017-03022-2
2. https://stanfordhealthcare.org/doctors/s/david-spiegel.html
3. Sonia Lyubomirsky, "The How of Happiness", Penguin Press HC, 2007.
4. Susan Nolen-Hoeksema, PhD, https://psychology.yale.edu/
5. https://nyulangone.org/doctors/1265983407/laura-e-price
6. https://weatherhead.case.edu/faculty/richard-boyatzis
7. https://www.rickhanson.net/

Notes

8. Grant, Adam, "Think Again: The Power of Knowing What You Don't Know", Viking, 2021

Behavior Myth #2 – Multitasking is Time Management

9. https://time.com/3855911/phone-addiction-digital-distraction/
10. https://www.fairfield.edu/media/fairfielduniversitywebsite/documents/academic/base_group_2.pdf.; Carol Leaf, "Switch On Your Brain", Baker Books, Michigan, 2013
11. https://news.stanford.edu/news/2009/august24/multitask-research-study-082409.html
12. Beck, J.S. (2011). Cognitive Behavioral Therapy: Basics and Beyond 2nd Ed. New York: The Guilford Press

Behavior Myth #3 – *Feedback is Criticism*

13. Jack Zenger and Joseph Folkman, Speed: How Leaders Accelerate Successful Execution (McGraw Hill, 2016); https://hbr.org/2013/12/overcoming-feedback-phobia-take-the-first-step
14. Harvard Business Review, April 2003, Retrieved from https://hbr.org/2003/04/fear-of-feedback.

Behavior Myth #4 - Work and Life Must Balance

15. Stewart Friedman, Total Leadership, Harvard Business Review Press, 2008
16. https://www.dol.gov/general/topic/workhours/flexibleschedules
17. Peterson, C., Park, N., Hall, N., & Seligman, M. E. P. (2009). Zest and work. Journal of Organizational Behavior, 30, 161-172
18. https://michiganross.umich.edu/rtia-articles/study-learning-something-new-could-help-reduce-stress
19. Adapted from Addicted to Busy, Your Blueprint for Burnout Preventing by Paula Davis-Laack, JD, MAPP

Chapter 6. Renovating to Realize Values: The Guiding Foundation

1. Koteinikov, Vadim (2008). "Values-Based Leadership: Energizing Employees to Pursue a Common Goal Using a Set of Shared Values.";
http://www.1000ventures.com/business_guide/crosscuttings/leadership_values-_based.html
2. https://www.ncbi.nlm.nih.gov/pmc/?term=articles+ethics+and+values
3. Wood, K. (2013). The lost art of introspection: Why you must master yourself.
https://themighty.com/topic/mental-health/study-how-many-thoughts-per-day

Chapter 7. Renovating to Realize Vision: What You Expect to See

1. Story retrieved from Dr. Myles Munroe, The Principles and Power of Vision, Keys to Achieving Personal and Corporate Destiny, Whitaker House, 2003
2. https://hbr.org/2014/05/from-purpose-to-impact
3. Viktor Frankl, Man's Search for Meaning, Beacon Press, 1746
4. Dr. Myles Munroe, The Principles and Power of Vision, Keys to Achieving Personal and Corporate Destiny, Whitaker House, 2003
5. Rob-Jan de Jong, The Art of Leading by Looking Ahead, AMACOM, 2015
6. https://www.gltgolf.com/golf-blog/golf-psychology-blog/golf-psychology-pre-shot-routine-jack-nicklaus-and-visualization.html
7. https://www.researchgate.net/publication/228118007_Does_Mental_Practice_Enhance_Performance

8. Scripture taken from the New King James Version®. Copyright © 1982 by Thomas Nelson. Used by permission. All rights reserved.

Chapter 8. Renovating to Realize Voice: Appreciating Your Brand

1. Morsella, E., Bargh, J.A., & Gollwitzer, P.M. (2009). Oxford Handbook of Human Action. New York, NY: Oxford University Press, USA
2. Inc. Real Talk, Simon Sinek on How Much Transparency is Enough, Retrieved from https://www.inc.com/video/simon-sinek-how-much-transparency-is-too-much.html
3. Brown, B. (2015). Daring Greatly: How the Courage to be Vulnerable Transforms the Way We Live, Love, Parent, and Lead. Avery
4. Martin Lanik, The Leader Habit: Master the Skills You Need to Lead--in Just Minutes a Day, AMACOM, 2018
5. http://www.ceebl.manchester.ac.uk/events/archive/aligningcollaborativelearning/Johnson_Johnson.pdf
6. https://www.psychologytoday.com/us/blog/the-good-life/201006/gratitude-letting-other-people-know-they-matter-benefits-us

Chapter 9. Rebuilding With Signature Strengths: Strength-Centered Leadership

1. Ito, T. A., Larsen, J. T., Smith, N. K., & Cacioppo, J. T. (1998). Negative information weighs more heavily on the brain: The negativity bias in evaluative categorizations — Journal of personality and social psychology, 75(4), 887.
2. Baumeister, R., Bratslavsky, E, Finkenaur, C., & Vohs, K.D. "Bad is Stronger than Good." Review of General Psychology, 5, 4, 323-370., 2001
3. Buckingham, M., and Clifton, D.O., The Strengths Revolution. Gallup Business Journal, 2001. https://news.gallup.com/businessjournal/547/Strengths-Revolution.aspx. Harter, J., Taking Feedback to the Bottom Line. Gallup Business Journal, 2001; https://news.gallup.com/businessjournal/814/taking-feedback-bottom-line.aspx;
4. Higgins, E.T. (1998). Promotion and prevention: Regulatory focus as a motivational principle, Advances in Experimental Social Psychology, 30, 1-46
5. Seligman, M. E. P., Steen, T. A., Park, N., & Peterson, C. (2005). Positive psychology progress: Empirical validation of interventions. American Psychologist, 60, 410–421
6. Niemiec, R. M. Character strengths interventions: A field-guide for practitioners. Boston: Hogrefe, (2018)
7. Mackie, D. (2014). The effectiveness of strength-based executive coaching in enhancing full range leadership development: A controlled study. Consulting Psychology Journal: Practice and Research, 66(2), 118–137

Chapter 10. Rebuilding With Emotional Resilience: Energized Leadership

1. The Resilient Factor: 7 Keys to Finding Your Inner Strength and Overcoming Life's Hurdles, 2002.
2. Youssef, C. M., & Luthans, F. (2007). Positive organizational behavior in the workplace: The impact of hope, optimism, and resilience. Journal of Management 33, 774-800. doi:10.1177/0149206307305562

Notes

3. McDonald, G., Jackson, D., Wilkes, L., & Vickers, M. H. (2012). A work-based educational intervention to support the development of personal resilience in nurses and midwives. Nurse Education Today, 32, 378-384
4. Haskell, W. L., Lee, I. M., Pate, R. R., Powell, K. E., Blair, S. N., Franklin, B. A., et al. (2007). Physical activity and public health: updated recommendation for adults from the American College of Sports Medicine and the American Heart Association. Med. Sci. Sports Exerc. 39, 1423–1434. doi: 10.1249/mss.0b013e3180616b27
5. Dr. Harry Barry, Emotional Resilience: How To Safeguard Your Mental Health, Orion Spring, 2018

Chapter 11. Rebuilding With Smart Habits: Functional Leadership

1. Neal, D.T., Wood, W., and Jeffery M., and Quinn, J.M. (2006). "Habits—A Repeat Performance." Current Directions in Psychology Science 15, 4, 198-202
2. James, W. (1899). "The Laws of Habit." https://www.uky.edu/~eushe2/Pajares/tt8.html
3. Wiley Online Library at https://onlinelibrary.wiley.com/doi/abs/10.1002/ejsp.674
4. Representation of the habit loop popularized by Charles Duhigg's book, The Power of Habit: Why We Do What We Do in Life and Business, Random House, 2014
5. Cialdini, R., Pre-Suasion, Simon & Schuster, New York, 2016

Chapter 12. Recharging the Business of Wellbeing: Conscious Leadership

1. Ryan, R. M., & Deci, E. L. (2001). On happiness and human potentials: A review of research on hedonic and eudaimonic wellbeing. Annual Review of Psychology, 52(1), 141-166
2. ScienceDirect Journal, Retrieved from https://www.sciencedirect.com/topics/psychology/flow-theory
3. https://www.fastcompany.com/90388635/the-reason-behind-the-need-to-be-busy
4. https://www.bfrb.org/index.php?option=com_content&view=article&id=23&Itemid=36
5. Manber, R., Bootzin, R.R., Acebo, C., & Carskadon, M.A., (1996), The effects of regularizing sleep-wake schedules on daytime sleepiness, Sleep, 19(5), 432-441
6. Sleepy drivers as dangerous as drunk ones. https://foxnews.com/health/2012/05/31/study-sleepy-drivers-equally-as-dangerous-as-drunken-drivers/
7. https://www.newscientist.com/article/mg23631470-600-wake-up-call-how-a-lack-of-sleep-can-cause-alzheimers/
8. American Psychological Association, 2014, Journal of Experimental Psychology. Give Your Ideas Some Legs: The Positive Effect of Walking on Creative Thinking. https://www.apa.org/pubs/journals/releases/xlm-a0036577.pdf
9. https://www.heart.org/en/healthy-living/fitness/fitness-basics/aha-recs-for-physical-activity-in-adults
10. Friedman, R. (2014). What you eat affects your productivity, Ognite80 https://www.ignite80.com/articles/2016/9/28/what-you-eat-affects-your-productivity
11. Ovadia, P., Stay Off My Operating Table, Ovadia Heart Health, 2021
12. https://pubmed.ncbi.nlm.nih.gov/28044281/
13. https://bjsm.bmj.com/content/48/12/973

14. Cleary, M., Schafer, C., McLean, L., & Visentin, D. C. (2020). Mental health and wellbeing in the health workplace. Issues in Mental Health Nursing, 41(2), 172–175
15. https://profiles.stanford.edu/david-spiegel?tab=publications
https://www.nbcnews.com/better/health/your-brain-prayer-meditation-ncna812376
16. Newberg, A., Waldman, M., Words Can Change Your Brain, The Penguin Group, 2013

Chapter 13. Recharging With Gratitude: Supportive Leadership

1. https://hbr.org/2011/02/secrets-of-positive-feedback
2. https://www.workhuman.com/resources/research-reports/how-the-great-resignation-will-shape-hr-and-the-future-of-work
3. Emmons, R.A., Crumpler, C.A. (2000). Gratitude as a human strength: Appraising the evidence. Journal of Social and Clinical Psychology 19(1), 56-69
4. McCullough, M.E., Emmons, R.A., Tsang, J.A. (2002). The grateful disposition: A conceptual and empirical topography. Journal of Personality and Social Psychology 82(1), 112-127
5. https://www.oxfordhandbooks.com/view/10.1093/oxfordhb/9780195187243.001.0001/oxfordhb-9780195187243-e-041, The Oxford Handbook Online
6. Grant, A. M., & Gino, F. (2010). A little thanks goes a long way: Explaining why gratitude expressions motivate prosocial behavior. Journal of Personality and Social Psychology, 98(6), 946–955. https://doi.org/10.1037/a0017935
7. https://www.forbes.com/sites/erikaandersen/2013/11/27/how-feeling-grateful-can-make-you-more-successful/?sh=5967fdc42de7
8. https://www.prnewswire.com/news-releases/new-bersin--associates-research-shows-organizations-that-excel-at-employee-recognition-are-12-times-more-likely-to-generate-strong-business-results-177627921.html
9. https://www.glassdoor.com/employers/blog/employers-to-retain-half-of-their-employees-longer-if-bosses-showed-more-appreciation-glassdoor-survey/?_cf_chl_jschl_tk_=a4rjrCyUzwwqE.20D2jeva1akGEhmneCFL5.h_rXjfo-1639521570-0-gaNycGzNBv0
10. https://hbr.org/podcast/2013/11/the-big-benefits-of-a-little-t
11. Davidai, S., & Gilovich, T. (2016). The headwinds/tailwinds asymmetry: An availability bias in assessments of barriers and blessings. Journal of Personality and Social Psychology, 111(6), 835-851
12. Mikoski, G.S. (2011). On gratitude. Theology Today, 67, 387-390

ABOUT DR. DEANA

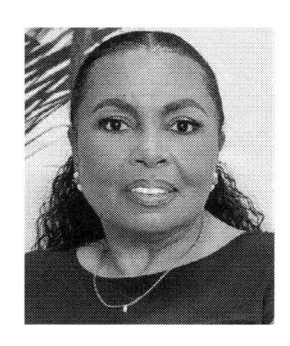

Dr. Deana earned her PhD with honors in Theological Psychology from Chesapeake Bible College with the focus on behavioral application. She continued to explore applied positive psychology, the science of wellbeing and human flourishing as a postdoctoral student at The Flourishing Center based in New York City. Dr. Deana is also an award-winning author of *Designing for the King*.

She established Dr. Deana, Inc., a boutique consultancy, dedicated to increasing the flourishing of individuals, organizations, and communities. She maintains a private executive consulting practice under the Lead2Flourish theme.

Her individual and group consulting clients include leaders from The NYC Office of Senior Court Attorneys, Johnsons Controls, Harvard Medical School, Weichert Realtors, SAFM, Temple University, Maryland Department of Labor, Asplundh, TechTown Detroit, Macy's, and others. She visited as a recurring guest lecturer at Temple University and was invited to keynote and teach in South Africa, Nigeria, London, and New Delhi, India.

Dr. Deana authored performance wellbeing essays for the Library of Professional Coaching and is a contributing writer at CEOWORLD Magazine. She continues to explore the science of human behavior and executive wellbeing to better understand what accounts for the good things that people do, and to help explain the bad things that sometimes occur.

Learn more about her at **DrDeana.com**.

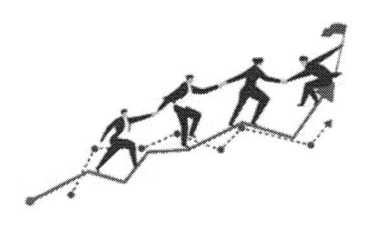

Notes:
- Subconscious contains insecurities that stem from childhood experiences.
- In an effort to protect ourselves from pain, we are triggered to protect threats to our Ego & act out with hostility, fear, anger & resentment to whatever or whomever is a threat to our EGO.

- Limiting Beliefs & UNCONSCIOUS UNPRODUCTIVE BEHAVIORS

- Respond vs React: Lead 2 Flourish requires a conscious effort to RESPOND to life instead of unconsciously REACTING to it.

- Our life is what our thoughts make it. p. 37

- p. 41 - Intentionally meditate on honorable, wholesome, lovely, right, admirable experiences. Then positive neurons will fire up for positive thinking - 10 minutes a day for at least 21 days. Intentional meditation on positive experiences wires healthy new thoughts deep into brain. Your brain shapes your world. p. 42

- Forgiveness - p. 42-43
- Designing a Plan p. 44
- Analysis Paralysis p. 48 — Paul

- p. 50-51 — Negative Ruminating about Paul & Gina what could happen in future. Negative Bias - dwelling on past negatives makes pessimism & clouds our creativity

Negativity Bias & Overthinking pp 52-55
Excavating the overthinking Mindset

R = recognize why
A = Assess accuracy of thinking
M = Make Ammendments - Modify thinking - REFRAME
B = Bright side: See & Savor the Bright Side - 20-30 sec on your reframed thought

My words: Terminal Negativity

Behavior myths & Misinformation: p. 46-79
1. Overthinking [BAD]
2. Multi-tasking is TIME MANAGEMENT - NO (= task switching)

Recognize task switching & how to undo it. p. 57 on
1. Recognize & be self aware.
2. Prioritize & make energy intensive - 20/80 rule. Do the 20% vital activities when you are FRESH - Do ONE at a time!
3. Simplify the complex & complicated. Do the difficult Before the easy. Put info in chunks
4. Catch yourself task switching
5. Center on focus time. 6. Leverage private time prefrontal cortex needs quiet time to assimilate info to be creative and harness memory, intellectual ability, & memory.

FAT THINKER - Think w/ Flexibility, Accuracy Thoroughly. Flexibly, accurately, thoroughly.

3. Feedback is criticism - Fear of Feedback
   Its how you frame it!! p. 66
4. Principles of undoing FEEDBACK PHOBIA
   1. Reframe the feedback to a Positive
   2. Reflect on it
   3. Restructure it.

#[4] Myth: Work & Life must Balance

Made in the USA
Columbia, SC
25 February 2023

eeb4fd1a-cf96-4b34-b24d-e9a5ea93e058R01